The Paleo Way: The Beginners Guide to Paleo

Secrets to Weight Loss, Eating Healthy, Naturally Fight Disease, Boost Your Energy and Improve Your Life

Recipes Included

Copyright 2019 ©

All Right Reserved
By Kiril Valtchev

DISCLAIMER

No part of this publication may be reproduced, stored in a retrieval system or transmitted in any form by any means, electronic, mechanical, photocopying, recording, scanning or otherwise, except as permitted under Section 107 or 108 of the 1976 United States Copyright Act, without prior written permission of the Publisher.

Limit of Liability/ Disclaimer of Warranty: While the publisher and author have used their best efforts in preparing this book, they make no representations or warranties with respect to the accuracy or completeness of the contents of this book and specifically disclaim any implied warranties of merchantability or fitness for a particular purpose.

No warranty may be created or extended by sales representatives or written sales materials. The information contained here is strictly for entertainment and information purposes only.

TABLE OF CONTENTS

INTRODUCTION

Paleo was developed millions of years ago and it is commonly referred to as the **"caveman diet"**. The diet is based on foods that were presumed to have been consumed by humans in the Paleolithic era.

During the Paleolithic era, people ate fish, fresh meat, fruits, and vegetables, along with other natural foods. A good wholesome Paleo way of eating.

People from the cavemen era had a healthier immune system, more energy, and better sleeping habits. They also had better weight control due to eating naturally fresh foods. The type of work they did in search for food and shelter to survive also contributed to their healthy lifestyle. Some of the benefits that you can experience with the Paleo diet is increased energy, increased sex drive, smoother skin, weight loss, better performance and shorter recover time. You will also develop a stronger immune system over time. These health benefits come after a period of detoxification that Paleo provides.

The cavemen's diet was packed with all the natural vitamins and nutrients that the body needed. Paleo recipes have more calories, more protein for recovery, and also less fat. Just think of how extreme a caveman's life was if Paleo kept him in shape, just think of the benefits it can have in the present time.

The Paleo way helped the cavemen get and maintain their natural strength, weight, blood sugar levels, mind power, and stamina just like any healthy diet should. I mean how many diabetic cavemen have you ever read about?

Even though we have come a long way in the storage of our food, with chemicals like sodium nitrate, salt, aspartame and phenylalanine, our immune systems can be seriously sabotaged if we fail to moderate out intake of specific foods. These chemicals which are used in the preservation process and substitution of our food, are all fine in small doses, but many people fail to adequately control their portions. As a result they end up creating health problems for themselves and those around them.

All things in moderation. Right? Chemicals prolong the shelf life of food, but at what expense?

Some of these additives discussed have been linked to health problems such as serious brain lesions, seizure activity, and even tumors.

A good Paleo food list starts from the outside walls of your local grocery store or your local farmers market. A well balanced Paleo menu starts with home grown or organic foods. This is just the tip of the iceberg. The way the Paleo diet plan puts it all together is really the key. From Paleo snacks to Paleo meatloaf, the variety of foods will leave you wanting nothing in the taste and variety section of your meats.

You might think that you have to change your whole life. I am here to assure you that you don't ! You just have to be a little more diligent when you shop for your food and have the desire to create a healthier lifestyle for you and your family.

Now let's get started !

CHAPTER ONE

WHAT IS THE PALEO DIET?

The Paleo diet is a low sodium, low sugar, high protein diet. It aims to provide you with the best health, by eating foods that our early ancestors in the Paleolithic era ate. While the diet prioritizes health, it can also be a great diet for weight loss. It is designed to work with your genetics so you stay lean, strong and naturally energetic.

The diet is believed to be the best suited for humans because genes have changed an insignificant 1%, while our current lifestyles and diets have changed dramatically. The overall thinking behind the diet is to go back to what caveman ate, with only fresh foods that are free of chemicals. Back in those days, cavemen freshly picked their foods or they would hunt for animals and would eat them as is, without any kind of preservatives, flavorings or additives.

In the Paleolithic era there was no such thing as instant food or food with a long shelf life. These are recent inventions by mankind to make our lives easier. With that, however, comes the price of health and thus preservatives and additives are put into our food to make it last longer and taste "better". It's more than obvious that majority of food today is not natural and in recent years we have been known to consume it in amounts that are harmful to our health.

The Paleo diet was created to spare us from chemicals that are not health and also to provide us with foods that contain what our bodies need to survive and lose weight in a healthy manner. The cavemen lived without McDonalds and so can you.

Due to the high intake of protein in the Paleo diet, consistent exercise is strongly recommended. Remember, cavemen had to walk for miles to gather their food and they had to run to hunt. That is why alongside the Paleo diet you need to have a regular exercise regime. The amount of protein in the diet can provide you with enough energy to perform tasks that are labor intensive. The diet includes fruits and vegetables in order to provide the body with the required vitamins and nutrients. These two food groups are healthy and there are no limits on their consumption, just consume with conscious moderation. The more you eat of these food groups over foods that contain additives and chemicals the better it will be for your system. There will not be a need to take vitamins or supplements because you will be getting enough vitamins and nutrition through the foods in the diet.

This diet is low in sugar and sodium simply because too much salt or sugar in the body is not healthy long term. The cavemen did not have a lot of sugar or sodium in their diet because artificial sweeteners, sugar and salt did not exist the way they do today. There was no need for excessive additives. It was all about survival.

The Paleo diet is all about going back to the basics by eating meat, fresh fruit, fresh vegetables and avoiding all kinds of processed foods that were not available in the Paleolithic era.

If you are looking to lose weight, this is the diet for you. It can help you slim down because you will be eating enough of the right foods that your body will know what to do with and how to properly process it. In turn, you will exercise and that will encourage your body to use your protein to build muscle, burn fat and ultimately lose weight. The Paleo diet consists of foods that are found in nature and only in nature.

In a nutshell, the diet consists of:

- Meat
- Fish
- Vegetables
- Eggs
- Fruits
- Nuts
- Seeds
- Herbs
- Spices
- Healthy fats and oils

Foods that are excluded from the Paleo diet include:

- Grains
- Legumes
- Dairy

- Refined salt and sugar
- Processed oils
- Soft drinks
- Processed and artificial ingredients
- Veggie oils
- Margarine

If you read the label of any typical junk food item, you will find many of these ingredients:

BROWNIES – Grains, Dairy, Refined salt/sugar, processed oil

CANDY – Refined salt/sugar, artificial colorings and chemicals

BREAD – Grains, Refined salt/sugar, processed oils, artificial colorings and chemicals

PASTA – Grains, Refined salt/sugar, processed oil, artificial colorings and chemicals

Most Restaurant Food – Grains, legumes, Refined salt/sugar, processed oil, artificial colorings and chemicals

WHY THE PALEO DIET?

There are many reasons to switch over to the Paleo diet in place of the farm-food diet that is harming your bodily functions in both obvious and insidious ways. Weight loss is easy with a diet that is high in protein and low in sugar and carbohydrates, which is what the Paleo diet is.

Feeling lighter and more energetic, shedding food-related problems like allergies and digestive irritation, and prolonging your life by reducing the chances of developing serious conditions like diabetes and heart diseases.

Our ancient forebears' had only high quality, low fat protein available to them. Saturated fats are not correctly metabolized by our bodies and therefore should be avoided. Sugar and salt as additives are also fully avoided when on the Paleo diet.

You can shake off persistent food-generated allergies by eating the foods that make the Paleo diet what it is, healthy. Gluten and casein are two substances introduced to our diet by the ill-advised choices of agriculture, to which our bodies respond with a variety of problems.

Paleo will greatly boost your chances of staying as healthy and as fit as our ancestors, rather than the overweight, diabetic, allergy-ridden population that exists today.

CHEAP FOOD HARMS THE ENVIRONMENT AND OUR BODIES

The reason for the Paleo diet is simple, it works. Human beings are made to eat certain foods and avoid others. Just like the animal kingdom, animals have a specific diet and we're no different. We refer to an animal's diet as a means of classifying them.

Such as:

- Herbivore (plant eaters)
- Carnivore (meat eaters)
- Omnivore (both plant and meat)

Humans today are mostly carnivore (meat eaters) and moderately herbivore (plant eaters). The point is that we are made to eat and thrive on NATURAL FOODS found in NATURE.

When you process food through heat, chemical, or other means you are removing the nature. Some foods, such as grains, are not meant to be consumed in their raw state and most undergo major heat processing to be edible for human consumption. This is a sign that we are **NOT MEAT TO EAT THEM!** Perhaps that is why gluten and grains cause so many gut and health issues.

Let's have a quick recap so you can keep up:

No processed anything – Grains, Legumes, Flour, Rye, Barley, Candy, Cake, Buttered or Fried food, etc.

All Natural, Nothing Added – Meat, Seafood, Veggies, Fruit, Potatoes, Yams, Nuts/seeds.

HOW PALEO CAN HELP YOU LOSE WEIGHT AND AVOID OBESITY

The Paleo diet is designed to help you make the right food choices which will allow you to start losing weight naturally and also help you feel healthier and more energetic.

Furthermore, the foods that you consume on the Paleo diet are not addictive and will not leave you feeling hungry.

It is amazing how eating non-addictive foods, which are common in the modern-day diet, can make such a dramatic difference to your health and weight.

It is by no accident that over 60% of Americans are overweight and obese. If you happen to be part of that statistic, it's not too late to make a positive change to your diet.

If you get started on the Paleo diet now, you can begin to see improvements in your weight and health in a short amount of time. All the weight loss that you experience will be totally natural, health and will stay off for good.

TIPS FOR SUCCESSFUL WEIGHT LOSS ON THE PALEO DIET

1. Keep your food and diet simple

One of the reasons the Paleo diet is so effective for weight loss is due to its ability to help you reduce calorie intake without constantly monitoring them or avoiding them. Studies have proven that consuming simpler foods leads to eating less, which can help you lose weight without constantly thinking about it.

How can I keep my Paleo diet simple?

We all have an idea of what a healthy meal consists of. We simply need to focus on the basics of a health meal. Eat plenty of protein like meat or fish, healthy doses of non-starchy vegetables, whole foods, carbs from root vegetables or fruit, and healthy fat in moderation.

I won't lie, I love a delicious gourmet meal prepared by master chef as much as anyone, but it's important to note that you CAN prepare delicious Paleo recipes from the comfort of your own home. You can allow yourself to indulge from time to time, but it's important to stay the course of the Paleo diet if you want to experience the many benefits it can provide.

Just cook simple dishes that don't contain a ton of different flavoring or fatty oils. It will make your food preparation easier and you can actually save money.

2. Eat enough

People new to the Paleo diet or any diet alone, typically associate eating less with losing weight. This common misconception can cause you to selectively deprive your body of the calories and nutrients it needs in order to function properly and can cause mental stress. Reducing your calorie intake too much can lower your resting metabolic rate **(the number of calories you burn just living)**, which can cause weight loss to slow down or even go in reverse. Regardless of which diet you select, it should never be about starving yourself and constantly obsessing over food. Calorie intake does matter, but when it comes to losing weight, starving yourself is never the answer.

What makes the Paleo diet unique is that it is more satiating per single calorie than any other diet around. This can help you consume less food without having to fight hunger or constantly counting calories. I see people who obsess about calories when trying to lose weight, and most of them end up failing to get any noticeable results. Constantly restricting calories isn't a viable weight loss strategy, but naturally consuming less food without a conscious effort is key to healthy and sustainable weight loss. This way you can have meals that are delicious without counting calories, and naturally eat less than you would on a standard diet. This is one of the major reasons why the Paleo diet is the smartest choice for healthy weight loss than many of the other traditional diets out there. You aren't starving, you aren't stressing, you're simply living a more health conscious lifestyle.

3. Eat the right amount of carbs

Carbohydrates tolerance varies person to person, and I have witnessed people who do very well on a very low carb diet, while others become dysfunctional. Typically, the major reason is isolated to the amount and intensity of the particular exercise the person is doing. Many people who are in the process of losing weight try to do so with highly popular programs, such as Crossfit, P90x or some sort of yoga. In the process, they end up neglecting their carb intake or end up consuming too much.

The simple truth is you need carbs. You don't have to restrict your carb intake, you just have to find the right balance of carb intake that will match your workout regime.

Insufficient carb intake can cause fatigue and muscle breakdown if you're over exercising and not taking in enough carbs to balance your activity levels. If you ramp up your exercise levels, you need to make sure you are consuming an adequate amount of carbs to match it. I've seen many people remove carbs entirely, avoiding even the smallest amounts of healthy choices like sweet potatoes and fruit. Most of the time, this practice can be harmful to your health.

If you can only exercise a few times a week **(due to certain conditions or reasons)** you may find that following a lower carb diet **(10-15% of calories)** may help you lose weight more effectively.

If you're consistently active, have a physically demanding job, or have tried a low carb diet in the past without much success, you may find that a moderate carbohydrate intake can be more effective **(20-30% of calories)** in your weight loss journey.

4. Mobility

Prolonged periods of inactivity can reduce the benefits of an exercise program and slow down your weight loss. If you happen to work in an office, you have to make the conscious effort to get up and move. Sitting around for long periods of time can be mentally and physically exhausting.

Exercise by itself is not enough, you have to be consistently active throughout the day. You must create daily habits that will help you stay mobile and energetic.

Being consistently active throughout the day benefits your health and promotes fat loss and even reduces your chances of developing diseases.

5. Don't be on a solo mission

One of the most difficult parts about losing weight is doing it all on your own. You don't have to be on a solo mission in order to lose weight. People all around you are in the same boat.

Lifestyle changes without any social support is not only difficult, but usually tough to sustain. Having a strong support system of friends and family around to push you, or even join you, can greatly increase your success in any major lifestyle change, particularly the switch to Paleo. You can exchange recipes, workout plans, ideas and push each other to stay motivated throughout the journey.

6. Lifestyle adjustment, not just diet.

Losing weight and keeping it off is more than just exercise and diet. It is the conscious decision to make a lifestyle adjustment that will benefit your health for the long term.

For example, getting less sleep can make us hungrier, aggravated, and lead to stress. High levels of stress can cause us to eat more and store more fat, which can reduce our ability to lose weight and keep it off.

People with social support have a better ability to handle stress, and personal-efficacy.

Focus on managing your daily stress by using mind-body techniques like meditation or yoga. Planning ahead using prepared shopping lists and meal plans can help reduce the stress that comes along with starting a big lifestyle change. Engage with friends and family and get support in your weight loss efforts. By getting support from friends and family you are more likely to stick to your goals and hold yourself accountable.

HEALTH BENEFITS OF PALEO

Benefit #1| Healthy Cells

Majority of people don't know this, but every cell in your body is comprised of saturated and unsaturated fats. Your cells depend on a healthy balance of the two in order to properly send messages in and out.

The Paleo diet naturally provides a good balance of fats because it uses them in moderation while other diets limits one or the other. It is the natural balance in the Paleo diet that helps promote healthy cell production in your body.

Benefit #2| Healthy Brain Function

One of the most effective sources of protein and fat used by the Paleo diet comes from freshwater fish, preferably wild-caught salmon.

Salmon fat is full of omega 3 fatty acids which is lacking in the average diet. Omega 3 fatty acids contain DHA **(docosahexacnoic acid)** which is known to be good for the eyes, heart, and most importantly the brain development and function.

Polyunsaturated fatty acids, or commonly referred to as (PUFA's), omega-3 fatty acids help promote growth and development of the brain. Other sources of omega 3 fatty acids can be found in pasture-raised meats and eggs.

Benefit #3| Build Muscle, Burn Fat

The Paleo diet relies heavily on the consumption of animal meat and along with it comes high levels of protein. The protein is very anabolic and is used for building new cells and packing on muscle mass.

The concept is very simple. The more muscle mass you have, the better your metabolism will work. This is because muscles require energy to move around and in order to move bigger muscles you must store more energy in them. This allows your body to send energy to muscle cells instead of fat cells.

The Paleo diet helps to increase the production of muscles cells and at the same time helps to shrink fat cells in the body. As a result, any extra energy produced by the body will be converted to glycogen in your muscles instead of triglycerides in your fat cells. This process helps you put on muscle and reduce fat.

Due to different genetic makeup, some people will tend to have higher metabolic rates than others, but your muscle mass is very important to consider when determining your BMR **(Basal Metabolic Rate)**. Your BMR is used as an estimate of how many calories you would burn if you did nothing but rest for 24 hours. It is meant to represent the minimum amount of energy required to keep your body fully functioning. Muscle is more active and energy-demanding than fat, so if you have a higher percentage of muscle compared to fat, you will have a higher BMR.

Benefit #4| Improved Intestinal Health

Sugar and processed foods can cause inflammation and intestinal irritability that will leave your feeling sluggish and even aggravated at times. When you combine large amounts of processed foods with stress you can develop a condition known as "leaky gut syndrome". When this happens, your small intestine will become irritated and inflamed. Large spaces will begin to form between the cells of your intestinal wall and will allow bacteria, toxins and food to leak through. In order for your body to properly digest food, it has to stay in the digestive track until it's fully ready to be transported to your cells. Since you will be avoiding processed food and foods high in sugar while on the Paleo diet, you will experience less stomach aches. Your overall intestinal health will improve.

Benefit #5| Improved Sustainability

The consumption of pasture-raised meats and eggs is highly encouraged on the Paleo diet. This means that the animal meat you consume must come from animals who are able to freely roam in their natural environment and grow without being force fed.

In their natural habitat, chickens tend to follow cows around and eat the bugs and larvae that are found under the cow pies. As a result, the cow pie will break down which will fertilize the grass and cause it to grow. The cows will then consume the very grass they roam around. It creates a natural sustainability which is free of pesticides and other chemicals.

This natural diet and sustainability is great not only for the animals but will also serve you with the best nutrients and lean protein.

Benefit #6| Vitamins and Minerals

Eating root vegetables is highly encouraged on the Paleo diet. Veggies are a major part of the diet and it's important to consumer vegetables daily while on it. They are highly packed with fiber, potassium, vitamin A and vitamin C.

The best vegetables to eat on the Paleo diet include:

- Broccoli
- Kale
- Peppers
- Onions
- Carrots

Benefit #7| Limits Fructose Intake

Why is fructose consumption a cause for concern?

The human body digests fructose differently than other complex carbs. The Paleo diet is meant to limit the amount of fructose you consume or to only eat certain fruits that tend to be low in fructose. Excessive amounts of fructose can cause damage to the outer walls of your liver and lead to the development of fatty liver disease. Consuming too much fructose can cause other health related problems such as diabetes, obesity and heart disease.

Fruits with low amounts of fructose include:

- Kiwi
- Grapefruit
- Lemons and Limes
- Cantaloupe Melon
- Tomatoes

Fruits with high amounts of fructose include: **(Avoid or limit consumption)**

- Figs
- Mangos
- Grapes
- Cherries
- Pomegranates

Benefit #8| Improved Digestion

The Paleo diet believes you should focus on eating foods that you've adapted the ability to digest over thousands of years. The human body is best suited to consumed starchy foods and grass-fed beef. Our ancestors not only survived under these foods but were extremely healthy and active.

Fermented foods, ranging from sauerkraut to yogurt, are being recognized as having major benefits to your digestive health. They have been shown to help with allergies and weight loss.

Benefit #9| Less Instances of Allergies

The Paleo diet focuses on avoiding foods that are known to cause allergic reactions to most people. There are many people who are not able to properly digest seeds and dairy. The Paleo diet focuses on avoiding these types of foods in order to prevent and avoid allergic reactions.

People often criticize others on the Paleo diet and say that they do not consume whole grains. This is very inaccurate. The reality is that grains are not considered to be healthy. They are one of the simplest forms of carbs and tend to break down into sugar very quickly. This can cause a spike in your blood sugar and your insulin levels.

Benefit #10| Reduced Levels of Inflammation

Research has proven time and time again that inflammation is a leading factor towards the development of cardiovascular disease. A major benefit of the Paleo diet is that majority of the foods are anti-inflammatory. This will great reduce your chances of developing any major heart problems.

The diet focuses on consuming foods that are rich in omega-3 fatty acids such as salmon and pasture raised animals. Foods rich in omega-3 fatty acids tend to be anti-inflammatory.

Research has proven that a healthy balance of omega-3 fatty acids in your diet can reduce inflammation and lower your chances for developing heart disease, cancer and arthritis.

Benefit #11| Increased Energy

Nowadays people are guzzling caffeine and energy drinks by the gallon a week. They are looking to improve their energy, but instead they are hurting their bodies in the process. The reason people are looking for extra sources of energy is because their diets are not providing them with the proper sources of energy. I constantly see people chugging energy drinks like its water just to get a temporary boost in energy. Little do they know, they are causing extreme damage to their bodies and internal organs.

The average working-class individual might drink anywhere between 2-3 cups of coffee per day, loaded with sugar and dairy mil and then continue their downward spiral with fast food. This is a recipe for developing serious health problems.

With the Paleo diet you will not need to consume copious amounts of caffeine to stay alert and energized. That is the whole point of the diet. It is meant to provide you with a natural source of energy through the healthy foods included in the diet. With the Paleo diet, you are selective in your food choices with a purpose. To be healthy and energetic.

The foods consumed on the Paleo diet have a low glycemic index. The sugars in the foods are absorbed quickly and efficiently. They will no marinate in your intestinal tract until you are left feeling sick. As a result, you will avoid having a lag in energy which can commonly occur after consuming foods and liquids that are packed with sugar and carbs.

Benefit #12| Weight Loss

By default, the Paleo diet tends to be very low carb. By removing processed foods from your diet, you will dramatically reduce the amount of carbs you consume and as a result experience healthy weight loss.

A good strategy to control the effects of carbs on your body is to consume them around your workout regime. This way you can quickly burn them and avoid the buildup of fat that is often caused with consuming excessive amounts of carbs.

Benefit #13| Improved Insulin Sensitivity

If you consumed chocolate cake with every meal, for a period of six months, it is highly likely that you will slowly begin to dread the taste of it. The same goes for how you treat your body. When you consistently feed your body processed and cheap foods your body will begin to react negatively.

Your body needs a sufficient dose of energy, and when you push your body outside of its limits it will reject fuel and begin to store it as fat. If this continues to happen consistently, over time you will begin gaining weight and become sensitive to insulin. Your body will fail to recognize when your cells are full, and you can begin to develop health problems.

Once you begin your journey with the Paleo diet, even in the short term, you will experience improved BP and glucose tolerance, decreased levels of insulin secretion and improved insulin sensitivity. You will begin to feel the positive effects of the diet as soon as your first week.

Benefit #14| Reduced Risk of Developing Heart Disease

Not everyone is a fan of the Paleo diet, but at the end of the day its main goal is to help improve your health. It focuses on helping you avoid foods that are potentially harmful to your health. It makes it easy to avoid eating harmful foods by providing you with a simple blueprint, only eat foods that your ancestors ate.

This approach may not be ideal for everyone, but it has proven to be effective for people who chose to follow it. The diet ensures you only consume whole foods, and by doing so it reduces your risk for developing heart related diseases.

Benefit #15| Shrink Your Fat Cells

Most people aren't aware of the fact that their fat cells contract and expand based on their specific diet. A person who is lean doesn't have less fat cells, they simply have smaller sized cells.

In order to keep your fat cells small you must consume healthy fats and control your carb intake. Healthy fats are packed tightly together within your cells and available for energy if you are insulin sensitive.

Synergy creates energy. The Paleo diet naturally provides the foods that will help you pack on muscle and normalize your insulin sensitivity. Limiting your carb intake will ensure that your cells remain active and ready to burn fat.

Other benefits include:

- Increased and more stable energy levels
- Improved sleep
- Clearer skin and healthier looking hair
- Mental clarity

CHAPTER 2

HOW TO START YOUR PALEO DIET

Step 1: Kitchen Makeover

Many of us like to think that we are strong willed, but when the temptation of food begins to lurk around the corner, many of us quickly forget the goal and task at hand. Dieting is tough, there is no question about that. You might hear people saying that dieting is easy, but that is because they have adopted it as their lifestyle. In order to be truly healthy, you must make the conscious effort to adopt it as a lifestyle instead of a temporary experiment.

In order to adopt the Paleo diet as a lifestyle you must kick old eating habits to the curb. This should start with a kitchen makeover. I'm not talking about redesigning your kitchen, I'm talking about getting rid of the poisonous junk in your kitchen that is harming not only your health but polluting the environment.

Trust me, you can do this, and you do have the necessary willpower. You may not realize it, but you consciously use your willpower everyday in your life.

- Getting up to go to work everyday
- Forcing yourself to study for that dreadful exam
- Avoiding the pizza in the break room
- Meeting sales goals
- Not flirting with you sexy coworkers

The crazy thing to me is that people fail to use their willpower for the most important things in their life, their health. Not only do people constantly neglect their health, they often refuse to admit that they are. Be honest with yourself. It will help you not only change your habits but stick to your plans.

If there is junk food in your home, it will eventually get eaten. Unhealthy foods are usually easier and less time-consuming to prepare than healthier alternatives. Naturally when we are tired, we will turn to the alternative that is easy to prepare and satisfies our taste buds. Your goal should be to make it difficult for yourself to find harmful food in your kitchen. The most effective way is to throw all the junk food away.

Get a large garbage bin and start going through your kitchen. You need to throw away the junk food that is taking up space in your kitchen and simply replace it with the foods provided on our list. Trust me, you'll be more than glad you did.

Let's Get Started!

1. Grab a large black trash bag and prepare to toss unhealthy items in it.

2. Open your pantry and look for the following items:

- Chips
- Pretzels
- Chocolate
- Candy
- Baked goods/Hostess/Little Debbie
- Instant foods (cake mix, mashed potatoes, macaroni)
- Flavored nuts
- Cereal
- Breads/bagels/pasta
- Crackers
- Granola bars

3. Open your freezer and look for the following items:

- Ice cream
- Frozen dinners
- Hot dogs
- Cookie dough
- Candy/chocolate
- Waffles

4. Open your fridge and look for the following items:

- Milk
- Fruit juice

- Alcohol
- Any calorie beverage
- Sweetened yogurt, sweetened anything
- Processed meats (deli, prepackaged)
- Restaurant leftovers
- Margarine
- Breads, bagels, whole grains
- Peanut butter
- Condiments (BBQ, ketchup, salad dressings, cream cheese)

These lists do no include everything you should avoid, but they should server you as a good starting point. If you have trouble pronouncing some of the ingredients on your food packaging, you probably shouldn't be consuming it.

While you may think you are wasting food by throwing it away, you are gaining more life. Most of the chemicals and substances in your food can destroy your health over time. Once you clear out your kitchen you will fee like a new person, and since you have most likely thrown out majority of your food the next step is to visit your local grocery shop to begin your Paleo journey.

Step 2: Take a Trip to the Grocery Store

You have to eat right, and an empty kitchen isn't going to fix that. Now is the time to hit your local Whole Foods, Trader Joe's, or regular grocery store and get your Paleo on.

You can use your complete approved Paleo food list to help you decide which foods you should and shouldn't be purchasing. For the most part, stick to the outer layers of the grocery store. This is where you'll find majority of the wholesome foods like fresh veggies, fruit, and animal protein like grass-fed beef, lamb, and salmon and chicken.

Here's a good rule of thumb for you to follow when buying your food:

0 ingredients – you have a winner

1 ingredient – you're good

3 ingredients – you're pushing it

4 or more ingredients – forget about it

Quick tip: Not everything you purchase needs to be organic. Organic foods tend to be more expensive and that is obvious to most people. You don't have to only buy organic to experience the benefits of the Paleo diet. Be more conscious of the ingredients that your food contains before you end up purchasing it. Absolutely avoid any microwaveable foods. It is riddled with harmful chemicals.

Step 3: Learn to cook

You have cleared out your kitchen and loaded it back up with healthy Paleo foods. What's next? For many of us, the mere thought of cooking can be intimidating, but you don't need to be Gordon Ramsay in the kitchen to make delicious, healthy, Paleo-friendly meals. Cooking Paleo meals is much easier than cooking other meals since you will be using less ingredients. Here is a step by step process for prepping your first Paleo meal.

Start by:

Putting a little oil in a pan, usually 1 tablespoon for every 6 ounces of meat is ideal. Don't overdue the oil.

- Brown some meat in the oil
- Add in some spices
- Add in your veggies
- Cover it up, and let it sit. Check on it every 2-3 minutes

You plate should be covered mostly with veggies, with animal protein taking up about one-third of the plate, depending on your weight and activity level.

Focus on using the following oils while cooking:

- Olive Oil (use at lower heat)
- Almond Oil
- Coconut Oil

- Avocado oil

Avoid using the following oils while cooking as they can become toxic and rancid rather quickly:

- Canola Oil
- Sunflower Oil
- Soybean Oil
- Cottonseed Oil
- Corn Oil
- Safflower Oil

Quick tip: Stick to making quick and simple recipes first. You don't need to get complicated when preparing your first couple of meals. It is much easier to establish healthy eating habits if you simplify the cooking process.

Recipes can be confusing and time-consuming, so we suggest using the tip above, or choosing a small list of go to recipes and becoming an expert at preparing them.

Step 4: Exercise Consistently

Cavemen and women spent the majority of their time constantly moving around on their feet, hunting for the food, building shelters, running from predators, starting fires and so much more. They were constantly active because they had to survive.

A good portion of their time was spent walking from place to place in search of a safe cave for a good night's sleep. They didn't have the stresses of bills, kids and careers. They simply had to survive.

Your fitness regime doesn't have to be complicated, it needs to be consistent. You don't have to always lift weights and run. You can use body weight to start building strength and endurance, and to increase your fat loss. Below are some ways you can stay active without having to constantly force yourself to go to the gym:

- Walk your dog around the neighborhood
- Ride your bike

- Join a local athletic team (indoor basketball, dodgeball, etc.)
- Mow the lawn
- Do some gardening
- Go for a swim

There are so many different ways to stay active that I could write a whole book about it. You just have to find ways to stay consistently active. You can't just diet and sit on your ass and watch re-runs of t.v. shows and expect life changing results. It doesn't work like that.

Quick tip: Force yourself to become more active in your daily routine by parking farther away from places you visit, taking the stairs, and jogging to get the mail.

Step 5: Get Some Rest

This is often an under looked topic. Sleep is extremely important for good health and mental stability. Your body needs time to recover. You'll need plenty of it in order to let your body recover from exercise and work. The benefits of good sleeping habits include:

- Improved performance in athletics
- Increased energy
- Improved mood and attitude
- Stronger immune system
- Higher tolerance for stress
- Enhanced memory and mental focus
- Decreased risk of obesity, heart disease, and type 2 diabetes

Let's check out some tips that will help you get a better night's sleep.

Limit the amount of television you watch or time you spend in front of a computer. The light and noise interfere with the deep and rejuvenating level of sleep required for ultimate health and energy. Cavemen didn't have cable, internet or cell phones to keep them up. They had dark caves.

Use dark curtains or blinds if street lamps or outside light tends to illuminate your bedroom at night. This will help you get deeper and longer sleep and you won't be constantly waking up in the middle of the night.

Your sleep cycle is disrupted when you're too warm or too hot. Most people have trouble sleeping when it becomes too hot. You want to sleep in a room that is cool enough. You don't need it to be freezing in there. My suggestion is to buy a fan.

Try sticking to a consistent sleep schedule. Sticking to a consistent sleep schedule will work wonders for your health. You will also have more energy throughout the day if your body gets used to having good sleeping patterns.

Take naps during the day from time to time. Naps can significantly improve your energy, stress levels and overall health.

Some things to watch out for:

If you're thinking about starting the Paleo lifestyle, the first two weeks may be a bit difficult for you to adjust to. During the first two weeks, your body id adjusting and cleansing itself, getting rid of toxins, and transitioning from being a sugar burner to a fat burner. During this period, you may experience slight fatigue and sugar cravings. You may get backlash from family members and friends about your new lifestyle. Don't let them discourage you. Most people like to scrutinize topics that are foreign to them. Yes, change can be daunting to most people, but without change how do you expect to see any progress?

Remember to focus on the three things below when first getting started.

1. Remember what you can eat, and not what you can't

When you tell people what you are not allowed to eat, they often begin to judge you, since they are most likely eating the foods you can't. It can come off as pretentious if you are judging them for choosing to eat differently than you. This is exactly the thing you are trying to avoid from happening to you, so don't judge others if they don't decide to conform to your lifestyle.

2. Focus on the results

Let the results do the talking. When the fat starts coming off, your energy will be naturally sustainable and healthy. You must focus on the long term-benefits and results of the Paleo diet. There will be hurdles in the beginning, but consistently focusing on the end results will keep you going.

3. Focus on consistency

There are tons of fantastic resources available to help you learn as much as possible about the Paleo diet. Continue to learn after you get through this book so that you can help others who may benefit the same way you will. When those interested in it start asking you questions, you will be well informed with information that they can also take advantage of.

TIPS FOR STARTING THE PALEO DIET

It was interesting to see how many people give conflicting pieces of advice about the Paleo diet. It just goes to show that there's no one right way to do the Paleo diet. It will vary person to person. Something that works for you won't necessarily work for someone else. Now go out there and get started!

Getting Started

- Pace yourself. (Take things at a steady pace, you don't need to overwhelm yourself)
- Get rid of food groups one by one (sugars, then dairy, wheat, beans and legumes)
- Jump in and cut out all the bad stuff progressively. (The 60 Day Challenge is a great way to do this.)
- Start by making your snacks Paleo, then transition to dinner, lunch, and then breakfast. You can also start replacing one meal per week with a Paleo meal instead.
- Transition slowly by no longer buying the bad stuff and eating what's left in your house until it's all gone.
- Do your research (Really decide if you want to go Paleo)

- Plan out your meals for the first two weeks
- Ger your family on board

The Mentality

- Don't just think of it as the "Paleo diet", think of it as a lifestyle adjustment. You want the change to be permanent and not just a temporary try.
- Instead of thinking about the commitment and lifestyle change, focus on the rewards the chang will bring.
- Don't start cheating but reward yourself from time to time.
- If you fall off the wagon, hop right back on and continue with the diet.
- Read motivational material to help you stick to the diet and take time to develop a disciplined approach.
- Be aware that the longer you stick to it the easier it gets. Don't overcomplicated the diet, keep it simple. It's meant to be simple, but effective.
- Keep your eyes on the prize.
- Be patient. Rome wasn't built in a day. This will be a process and a long-term journey.

Making Paleo Easy

- Invest in a deep freezer so that you can stock up meat during sales and discount periods.
- Plan on making boiled ages as your go to breakfast meal.
- During your weekends, plan your meals, and prepare enough food to last you a few days or a whole week.
- Find a go to snack for when you're hungry but unable to cook.
- Prepare snacks ahead of time
- Pack food when you leave the house.
- Always plan two meals ahead so that you have the ingredients you need on hand.
- Know when to reward yourself.
- Keep a list of acceptable foods on the fridge and use it as a list of options when you want to snack.
- **No fast food, ever !!!**

- Eat the way that suits you, not the way someone else thinks you should eat.
- Stay hydrated by drinking lots of water.

Making Paleo Fun

- Make your own Paleo-friendly ketchup.
- Eat bacon and dark chocolate in moderation to make giving up junk food easier.
- Have small cheat days in order to reward yourself.
- Use Frank's Red-Hot Sauce
- Snack on almonds and other healthy nuts.
- If you have a sweet tooth, check out some of our desert recipes we included.
- Use fresh herbs when preparing your food.
- Find Paleo versions of recipes you are used to making.
- Adjust recipes to make them suit you.

PALEO FOOD LIST: WHAT YOU CAN AND CAN" T EAT ON THE PALEO DIET

The Paleo diet tends to be very controversial, mainly for its basis in a few debatable theories. The most important of which being that modern humans are adapted to the diet of early humans from the Paleolithic era, and that our genetics have not changed much since then. As such, the Paleo diet consists of foods that would have been naturally accessible to early humans, ruling out all processed foods and other products obtained only through technologically advanced agricultural means.

So, what is left for people to eat on the Paleo diet in our era? We have come up with an extensive list of approved and disapproved foods for the diet. The more closely you stick to the foods on the list, the more benefits you will experience from going Paleo.

Five Food Groups vs. Paleo Food List

Most of us have learned as early as elementary school about the five major food groups and how they are essential to a healthy and well-balanced diet. This is common knowledge for most people.

The five food groups consist of the following:

- Protein
- Dairy
- Fruit
- Vegetables
- Grains

The five major food groups won't apply to you when you are on the Paleo diet since the diet focuses on avoiding grains, dairy and fruit that is high in fructose. The Paleo diet focuses primarily on protein, vegetables and fruits that are low in fructose.

The caveman did not eat dairy or grains because they were living in an era where modern agriculture didn't exist. Milking animals was out of the question, and milling grains was not even a concept during that time. The only things on the table was meat, fruit, vegetable and some health portions of seeds and nuts.

PALEO FOOD LIST: APPROVED FOODS

People following the Paleo diet are allowed to eat Paleo approved meats, vegetables, fruits, nuts, oil and fats. Let's begin with the meats. Don't worry, your options are bigger than you think.

Paleo Approved Meat

You have plenty of options to choose from when it comes to Paleo approved meats, as long as the meat is fresh and unprocessed. If it's meat you could have caught, killed and prepared in the wild, without the use of any chemicals, you are good: These include:

- Bacon

- Bear (yes, some people actually eat bear meat)
- Beef jerky
- Bison
- Bison jerky
- Bison ribeye
- Bison sirloin
- Bison steaks
- Buffalo
- Chicken breast
- Chicken leg
- Chicken thigh
- Chicken wings
- Chuck steak
- Clams
- Elk
- Emu
- Goat
- Goose
- Grass fed beef
- Ground beef
- Lamb chops
- Lamb rack
- Lean veal
- New York steak
- Ostrich
- Pheasant
- Pork
- Pork chops
- Pork tenderloin
- Poultry
- Quail
- Rabbit
- Reindeer
- Turkey
- Venison steaks
- Wild boar

Paleo Approved Fish and Seafood

Fish is another great source of protein because it's low in fat and loaded full of omega-3 fatty acids. These include:

- Bass
- Clams
- Crab
- Crawfish
- Halibut
- Lobster
- Mackerel
- Oysters
- Red Snapper
- Salmon
- Sardines
- Scallops
- Shark
- Shrimp
- Sunfish
- Swordfish
- Tilapia
- Trout
- Tuna
- Walleye

Paleo Approved Veggies

Almost all vegetables are allowed in the Paleo diet, except for legumes and beans, which are sometimes considered vegetables, but many of which are technically grains. The best veggies to eat on the Paleo diet are root vegetables. The variety of vegetables which you can eat is big. These include:

- Acorn squash
- Artichoke
- Artichoke hearts
- Avocado
- Beets

- Broccoli
- Brussels sprouts
- Butternut squash
- Cabbage
- Cantaloupe
- Carrots
- Cauliflower
- Celery
- Chives
- Cilantro
- Cucumber
- Dill
- Eggplant
- Garlic
- Green Onions
- Kale
- Lettuce
- Mushrooms
- Onions
- Parsley
- Parsnip
- Peppers
- Pumpkin
- Radish
- Shallot
- Spinach
- Sweet Potatoes
- Yam
- Zucchini

Paleo Approved Fruit

People on the Paleo diet should consume about one to three helpings of fruit a day, but do not go overboard. Yes, fruit is healthy and packed with good nutrients, but certain fruits can be high in fructose.

While on the diet, you will be avoiding fruits that are high in fructose. Stick to the fruits on our list and you will be fine. You still don't want to consume too much sugar though, even naturally. Put a priority on vegetables over fruit, but when you do eat fruit, below is a good list to follow:

- Apples
- Bananas
- Blackberries
- Cantaloupe
- Figs
- Grapes
- Guava
- Lemon
- Lime
- Lychee
- Mango
- Oranges
- Papaya
- Peaches
- Pineapple
- Plums
- Raspberries
- Strawberries
- Tangerine
- Watermelon

If you find it difficult to regularly get healthy portions of fruits and vegetables during the day, consider preparing in the mornings as starter snack or even as an addition to your breakfast. Invest in a juicer and being making healthy smoothies that are packed with fruits and vegetables. It will help you get your daily dose of fruits and vegetables.

Paleo Approved Nuts

Nuts and seeds are a good supplemental source of protein, but they tend to be high in fat. It can be tough to figure out which nuts and seeds are Paleo friendly.

For instance, some foods commonly referred to as nuts – such as peanuts- are legumes, which are a type of grain disapproved by the Paleo diet. Below is a list of the nuts you can eat on the Paleo diet:

- Almonds
- Cashews
- Hazelnuts
- Macadamia nuts
- Pecans
- Pine nuts
- Pumpkin seeds
- Sunflower seeds
- Walnuts

Paleo Approved Oils and Fats

Fat isn't terrible for your body if you consume it in moderation. As mentioned before, it's overly sugary, starchy foods like carbs that you want to avoid in excess. Fats are still necessary for the body to create energy. Plus, you need it if you want to cook. Below is a list of Paleo approved oils and fats:

- Avocado oil
- Coconut oil
- Macadamia oil
- Olive oil

Some people on the Paleo diet will consume grass fed butter, even though butter is a dairy product that is not part of the Paleo diet. It's a tough call, but if grass fed butter is too difficult to remove from your diet completely, then that's ultimately your choice to make.
There is no diet police that's going to come knocking on your door telling you that you're doing Paleo wrong, so have at it if you need to.

PALEO FOOD LIST: DISAPPROVED FOOD

Next, we have a guide to the foods that are not part of the conventional Paleo diet. The foods listed here should be completely avoided. If you have trouble avoiding majority of the foods on this list, you must focus on consuming them in moderation. Going Paleo isn't going to happen overnight for most people. If you still want to enjoy some of the foods on this list, you can. However, if you are planning to transition to Paleo, you must limit your consumption. Let's look at the foods you should be avoiding.

- Dairy products
- Sugary fruit juice
- Soda and other soft drinks
- Energy drinks
- Grains and legumes
- Processed meat
- Snack food
- Unnaturally salted food
- Candy
- Dairy
- Butter
- Cheese
- Cottage Cheese
- Cream Cheese
- Frozen yogurt
- Ice cream
- Milk
- Powdered milk
- Pudding
- Skim milk
- Yogurt

Fruit Juice

Remember, it's okay to juice fruits that are Paleo approved, but the Paleo diet doesn't allow sugary and processed fruit drinks that contain unnatural flavors, sweeteners, or enrichments. Below are juices you should avoid:

- Apple juice
- Cranberry juice
- Grape juice
- Mango juice
- Orange juice
- Soft Drinks

Soda is even worse than fruit juice, since it's a highly unnatural beverage made from carbonated water, and completed packed with high fructose corn syrup, sugar, and artificial sweeteners. Stay away from soda of all kinds! Let's look at some of your favorite sodas that you should avoid:

- ALL OF THEM

Energy Drinks

Energy drinks are even less Paleo than soda, and they should be completely avoided. Energy drinks are one of the most harmful products on the market. They are loaded with synthetic ingredients and chemicals that do nothing but deteriorate your insides. You should avoid all energy drinks. If you are not familiar with which ones see our list below:

- ALL OF THEM

Grains and Legumes

The most extensive list of unapproved Paleo diet foods are the grains, legumes, and associated products. These might be the most difficult to remove from your diet, but they are the most important to remove. They will have the biggest impact on your health. They are highly processed foods that are very unnatural and full of artificial additives that are harmful to your health if consumed in large quantities and long term. Take note, the following list is not all inclusive:

- Adzuki beans
- Beer
- Black beans
- Bread
- Cereals
- Chickpeas
- Corn
- Corn syrup
- Crackers
- Cream of wheat
- Fava beans
- Garbanzo beans
- High fructose corn syrup
- Kidney beans
- Lentils
- Lima beans
- Mung beans
- Oatmeal (can consume in healthy moderation)
- Pancakes
- Pasta
- Peanut butter
- Peanuts
- Peas
- Pinto beans
- Red beans
- Sandwiches
- Soybeans
- String beans
- Sugar snap peas
- Toast
- Tofu
- Wheat
- Wheat Thins
- White beans

Other foods and beverages like alcohol, candy, and processed meats like deli meat and spam speak for themselves.

A PALEO SHOPPING LIST FOR BEGINNERS

So, you're trying this whole Paleo diet for the first time. The last thing you need is to step foot into the grocery store with no clue what to buy. If frustration kicks in, so will the bread aisle. Stay calm and take a prepared Paleo shopping list with you the next time you head to the store. It's not everything on the Paleo-approved list, but it's the perfect start to this high-protein, low-carb, no-junk-food way of eating.

Be prepared, you will eat a ton of protein. Let's look at a sample shopping list. Don't be afraid to try something new if it looks foreign to you.

Meats

- Chicken
- Eggs
- Fish (Preferably Salmon)
- Pork
- Red meat
- Turkey
- Chicken sausage

Veggies

- Acorn squash
- Beets
- Bell peppers
- Broccoli
- Brussels sprouts (really good with bacon)
- Butternut squash
- Cabbage
- Carrots
- Cauliflower ** warning, may give you the farts**
- Celery
- Cucumber

- Mushrooms
- Leafy greens
- Onions
- Spaghetti squash
- Sweet potatoes
- Zucchini

Deserts/Fruits

- Apples
- Avocados
- Bananas
- Berries
- Cantaloupe
- Grapes
- Lemons
- Mango
- Pears
- Pineapples
- Tomatoes
- Watermelon

Snacks

- Almonds
- Cashews
- Hazelnuts
- Pumpkin seeds
- Sunflower seeds
- Walnuts
- Wine isn't on the list, but if you enjoy a nice Cabernet from time to time, have a little to reward yourself. Don't make it a daily routine though.
- Coffee
- Coconut water
- Club soda
- Kombucha
- Sparkling water
- Tea

CHAPTER 3

PREPARING TO GO PALEO

The Paleo diet has been gaining followers by the hundreds of thousands. Many people give credit to the low-carb, high-protein diet for their weight loss successes.

Before getting started on the diet, it is important to prepare yourself mentally for the foods you will need to cut out. You'll also need to stock up on some essentials both in terms of foods and kitchen equipment to make preparing to go Paleo easier and hassle-free.

Pre-cook your meals

On the Paleo diet, remember to moderate your intake of nuts and seeds as well as salt, and do not overdo it on the fruits. The diet will require planning and it is therefore essential to stock up on your vegetables, grass fed meat and lots of containers as you might be cooking enough food for the week or for lunches during the day. For people with a busy lifestyle, pre-cooking meals for the week will ensure that you do not revert to old habits of drive-ins and fast food.

Kitchen Essentials

When preparing your kitchen for your Paleo journey, you will need to get quality knives, particularly chef's and paring knives for all the slicing, dicing and chopping that you will be doing. Peelers, shears and knife sharpeners will also come in handy and will make quick work of the various ingredients you will be preparing for the various meals. Skillets, stockpots and saucepans will also become your best friends with this diet as well as gloves or mitts to ensure you will not be sautéing your fingers any time soon.

Wire racks and baking sheets will help keep your meals less fatty and oily which is a good thing not only nutrition-wise but also for the taste of the food. Tongs will help with the grilling and silicone spatulas will on only liven up your kitchen but are also heat-resistant and will not melt into your eggs as you turn them.

The Paleo diet is a healthy lifestyle change, and there are plenty of recipes available as well as large community out there that can help to ensure that you have nutritious and delicious meals while on the diet.

PREPARING YOUR MIND

Aggravating Factors

The pre-impact period of the Paleo diet can be split into two categories:

- **Threat:** Anger exists, some recognize and start acknowledging, while others don't recognize or don't accept and respond with denial or minimal acknowledgement.
- **Warning:** Everyone recognizes the danger and response is likely to be hyper-activity (lots of chatter, ideas and unhelpful suggestions, often leading to individual becoming very distracted).

The impact period is the emotional stage and has been shown to be statistically divided into three behavior groups:

- 10-20% of people are calm and fully aware of the transition and impact
- 75% react poorly and are unable to properly contain their emotions and physical responses
- 10-25% are off the wagon, often screaming and extremely irritable

This so-called recoil period follows the impact period, and depending on the individual, can last anywhere from a few hours to a few days. Typically, this is the time when people slowly being to normalize and rationale kicks back in.

Post-trauma stress of the diet can occur if the recoil period doesn't happen. In short, this is when individuals begin to fully understand the impact of whatever happened, and a wide range of emotions set in.

Sometimes we tend to react in survival situations due to an extreme event, but often we begin the progression because we are aware of the changes taking place and are fully embracing them. However, it is worth noting that we can experience some aggravation during the initial stages of the diet. Some of the most common aggravating factors you may experience when first getting started on the diet are:

- Short-term hunger
- Irratability
- Lack of concentration (varies person to person)
- Apathy
- Depression (varies person to person)
- Thirst, short-term and acute problem until fully adjusted
- Agitation
- Irrational behavior
- Fatigue

It's important to note that you may not experience any of these. The best way to handle the physical and psychological responses discussed above are:

- **Training** – Understanding your reactions, having the right approach and training are some of the most effective mitigation techniques to prevent and resolves these factors.
- **Motivation** – Have the will to stay motivated. Know what your end goal is with the diet. This will lead to overcoming the severe physical and psychological discomforts and allows you to create and achieve your present goals.
- **Discipline** – Staying consistent long term will have the biggest positive results to the diet. It will reinforce your goals and create a hopeful approach.
- **Acceptance** – Accepting your situation and responding with a positive outlook is key. This doesn't mean giving in to it but responding with rationale rather than doubt.
- Helping others – If you happen to be in a group situation look for 80-90% that need help with their psychological state.

We often don't think about how to prepare ourselves mentally when taking on a new challenge in life. Staying mentally prepared and focused is your number one solution to being consistent with any change.

Prepare both your mind and your body for the change and you will increase your odds of experiencing success.

TRANSITIONING TO PALEO

Making the transition to Paleo can be physically and mentally tough. The internet is full of excuses and bad experiences:

- I was too tired
- I was spending too much time in the kitchen
- Too many headaches

The diet is also equally full of positive reassurances:

- Everything is going according to plan
- I feel better already
- I'm seeing the pounds come right off

Each experience will vary person to person. The transition will be different for everyone depending on how serious they take the diet. The most important thing is to use a method that works for you.

In case you get lost in the process, remember the following.

Portions

Don't get caught up in overthinking your portions. You don't need to know everything before you start. It's not a problem if you mess up at the beginning. This will be a process and a learning experience. Take slow steps to transition as you learn more. Once Paleo eating becomes habitual for you (a few weeks to a few months), then you will have more time and energy to focus on becoming more proficient.

Transitioning to Paleo will force you to take on two different challenges at the same time:

- Getting fully educated on the diet and the process
- Making changes to your daily habits which will require a lot of planning, willpower, and energy.

Everyone Is Different

You need to focus on finding a transition strategy that works for you and your lifestyle. The process and experience of going Paleo will be entirely different for everyone. Just because something worked for your friend or colleague doesn't mean it will work for you.

Answer the following questions below to see specific recommendations which might speak to you.

- How do you prefer to make changes in your life?
- Do you live alone?
- Are you trying to lose weight with Paleo?
- Are you planning to do any difficult exercise while on Paleo?
- Are you on a special diet right now?

At the end of the day you have to be honest with yourself. Do you want to make the commitment to improve your health? It seems like an obvious answer, but most people fail to answer this question honestly.

There's a lot of misinformation about the transition process to Paleo.

Many people won't notice the typical side effects of the transition because they already practice a healthy diet or their body just doesn't react to it. But some people will experience physical symptoms ranging from headaches to digestive problems and exhaustion.

Large weight losses can release toxins stored in fat tissue. The weight loss won't start immediately, because it's directly proportional to the amount of fat tissue lost. If you see a very rapid 5-10 pound loss, it's almost certainly water weight and won't contain majority of these toxins. If you're experiencing detox symptoms from this process, the symptoms will slowly start appearing and continue at a relatively constant rate throughout the loss. Trust the process and you will experience positive results.

CHAPTER 4

PALEO MEAL PLANNING: Step by Step

Meal Planning Step 1: The Weekly Prep

When you eat Paleo, you will be cooking at home (a LOT) but one thing that can slow you down is preparing every single meal fresh, from scratch. By eating leftovers, you'll be able to reach into the fridge, grab and reheat a meal without having to start the process from step one.

Having a specific cook-up day is an important part of prepping your weekly meals. You'll need to set aside one day a week to do a big shopping trip and enough cooking to last you about a week. (Two to three hours will usually be enough). Pick a day where you don't have to work. If you're off on the weekend, you can use either Saturday or Sunday to do your meal prep.

With enough planning you'll be able to create meals for Monday through Friday. Then on the weekend you just repeat the process. A trip to the market and some weekend cooking. Adjust your cooking schedule to the days you have off. You will actually save money in the long run by prepping your meals because you won't be throwing as much food away.

My must-have tools for weekly prep:

- Programmable slow cooker
- Baking sheets for roasting vegetables
- Blender for sauces, soups and smoothies
- Containers to store your meals

Meal Planning Step 2: Create a prep sheet

This is the key to successful meal planning. Create a template that you categorize your meals by. This way, you keep the template and swap the recipes week to week so that you're taking some of the guesswork out.

Here's what I mean:

Monday:

Breakfast: Frittata, blueberries, cherry tomatoes

Lunch: Slow cooker chicken, roasted veggies, avocado

Dinner: Salad with grilled or pan-fried chicken, homemade dressing and nuts

Tuesday:

Breakfast: Hardboiled eggs, leftover slow cooker chicken, roasted sweet potato

Lunch: Stir fry, raw veggies, olives or coconut flakes

Dinner: Soup or stew, roasted squash, avocado

Wednesday:

Breakfast: Pan-fried chicken, veggies hash, homemade ranch

Lunch: Mixed salad with shredded pork, berries and avocado

Dinner: Tacos or enchiladas, fresh salsa and veggie juice

Thursday:

Breakfast: Egg muffins, fresh fruit, coconut flakes

Lunch: Leftover enchiladas from the previous day

Dinner: Out to eat

Friday:

Breakfast: Hardboiled eggs, smoked salmon with lemon, olives

Lunch: Salad with slow cooker chicken, homemade salad dressing

Dinner: Oven-baked meatballs and sauce with spaghetti squash, sautéed greens

Saturday:

Breakfast: Sweet potato hash, bacon and eggs

Lunch: Collard wraps, avocado and fruit

Dinner: Baked salmon with homemade sauce, fresh tomatoes

Sunday:

Breakfast: Forage for leftovers

Lunch: Lettuce-wrapped burgers and sweet potato fries

Dinner: Slow cooker curry with cauliflower rice

Leftovers will depend on how much you eat or if you want to prepare more meals.

Other Paleo Meal Planning Tips

Have Fun and Get Creative

You don't have to constantly cook for hours and wonder what your next meal is going to consist of. By mixing a variety of techniques, you can minimize your cooking time. Eating a mix of raw and cooked veggies will help.

Want healthy Paleo meal ideas?

Every week can include:

- Soups or stews
- Meatball soup
- Spiced Butternut squash soup
- Thai Coconut Soup
- Crock Pot Mocha-Rubbed Pot Roast
- Honey Mustard Crock Pot Spare Ribs
- Slow-Cooker Chocolate Chicken Mole
- Chicken Stir Fry
- Taco Salad with Creamy Cilantro Lime Dressing
- Baked egg dishes
- Breakfast sausage scotch eggs
- Paleo Carnitas Egg Muffins
- Hearty Spinach Beef Frittata
- Hardboiled eggs
- Vegetable hashes
- Apple Cinnamon Maple Bacon Sweet Potato Hash
- Simple Braised Root Veggies
- Roasted vegetables
- Rosemary Balsamic Butternut Squash
- Apple Cranberry Sweet Potato Bake
- Will's Yam Fries
- Sautéed vegetables
- Ratouille a la Claudette
- Cumin Coconut Chard
- Cabbage with apple and onion
- Raw salads or slaws
- Jicama Carrot slaw
- Watermelon Mojito Salad
- Grilled, pan-fried or baked meats/fish
- Pan-fired lemon chicken
- Mediterranean Turkey burgers
- Roasted Salsa Verde
- Roasted Butternut squash soup
- Paleo beef stew
- Oven baked meatballs

Next, we will look at some of the delicious breakfast, lunch and dinner recipes that you can used to get started on your Paleo journey.

CHAPTER 5

BREAKFAST MEAL RECIPES

Coconut Fat Bombs

Ingredients

- 1.5 cup of shredded coconut
- ½ cup coconut oil
- ½ cup of coconut butter or cream
- 1 tsp. vanilla extract (make sure there is no sugar)
- 1 pinch of sea salt

Top layer:

- ½ cup coconut oil
- ¼ cup almond butter
- ¼ cup cocoa powder
- 1 tbsp. honey
- ¼ cup walnuts (optional)

Instructions:

Step 1: Mix all the ingredients together in a large bowl or a food processor. If you are using solid fat, melt it down first and then add to the mixture.

Step 2: Begin to slowly form small to medium sized balls and the pour the mixture into a muffin pan or baking pan with tinfoil. You can shred some walnuts and add them into the mixture if you want.

Step 3: Once you have put the balls on the pan, put them in the refrigerator until the mixture solidifies. This should take 20-30 minutes.

These should be kept cold. One or two with a cup of black coffee makes for a delicious breakfast!

Quick Paleo Bread

Ingredients:

- 1 cup of creamy almond butter
- 3 eggs
- 1 tbsp. apple cider vinegar
- 1/2 tsp. of baking soda
- ¼ tsp. of salt
- 1 tsp. honey

Instructions:

Step 1: Preheat oven to 350 degrees F.

Step 2: Blend the almond butter and eggs until they have a smooth texture. Mix in the remaining ingredients.

Step 3: Stir the remaining ingredients until everything is well mixed and consistent.

Step 4: Put melted coconut oil on a bread pan and then pour the mixture onto the pan. Bake for 30-40 minutes until the bread becomes fluffy.

Paleo Pumpkin Muffins

Ingredients:

- 1.5 cups almond flour
- ¾ cup canned pumpkin
- 3-4 eggs, cage free
- 1 tsp. baking powder
- 1 tsp. baking soda
- 2 tsp. pumpkin pie spice
- 1 tbsp. almond butter
- 1 tbsp. sliced almonds or pumpkin seeds
- Pinch of sea salt

Instructions:

Step 1: Preheat oven to 350 degrees F.

Step 2: Cover the muffin tins with coconut oil. Mix all ingredients and pour into muffin tins.

Step 3: Bake for 25-30 minutes on the middle rack of the oven.

Step 4: Sprinkle nuts or seeds on top of muffins after removing them from the oven.

Beets and Berries Smoothie

Ingredients:

- 1 large frozen banana
- 2 cups frozen strawberries
- 1 medium sized avocado
- 1 large beet peeled and grated
- 1 cup almond milk

Instructions:

Put all the ingredients in a blender and blend until smooth and creamy and add cold water if necessary. Serve when it is nicely blended and consistent.

Liver Sausage and Eggs

Ingredients:

- ¾ pound group pork
- ½ pound ground beef
- ¼ pound ground beef liver
- 1 tbsp. maple syrup
- 1 tsp. dried sage
- ½ tsp. dried thyme
- ½ tsp. dried rosemary
- ½ tsp. sea salt
- ½ tsp. black pepper
- 2 tbsp. olive oil
- 4 large eggs (cage free)

Instructions:

Step 1: Combine the pork, beef, liver, maple syrup, seasonings, salt and pepper in a large bowl. Mix with your hands until well combined, and form into 2-inch patties.

Step 2: Heat the olive oil in a skillet and cook the patties until well browned and cooked through.

Step 3: Remove the sausages, add the remaining oil and fry the eggs to your liking. Serve with the sausages.

Green Smoothie Bowls

Ingredients:

Smoothie

- 1 medium sized avocado
- 3 medium sized frozen bananas
- 1 cup diced pineapple
- 2 cups chopped spinach or kale
- 2 tbsp. almond butter
- ½ cup unsweetened almond milk

Toppings

- ½ cup freshly sliced strawberries
- ½ cup chopped pecans
- ¼ cup shredded coconut
- 1 tbsp. toasted sesame seeds
- ¼ tsp. turmeric
- ¼ tsp. cinnamon

Instructions:

Step 1: Put the smoothie ingredients in a blender and blend until it is thick and creamy, adding a little water if necessary. Be careful not to add too much liquid, you want it to be thicker than a smoothie. Divide the mixture between bowls.

Step 2: Top with the toppings and serve with a spoon.

Ginger Turmeric Smoothie

Ingredients:

- 1 medium banana
- 1 cup dried pineapple
- 1 teaspoon freshly grated ginger
- ½ tsp. turmeric
- 1 medium sized lemon
- 1 cup coconut milk
- 1 cup of rice

Instructions:

Put all the ingredients in a blender and blend until smooth. Drink immediately or store in the fridge for a snack.

Coconut Lime Pancakes

Ingredients:

- ½ cup coconut
- 2 tsp. baking powder
- ¼ tsp. sea salt
- 1 cup almond flour
- 1 medium lime (juiced)
- 1 large egg (cage free)
- 2 tbsp. raw honey
- 1 cup coconut milk
- ¼ cup water
- 3 tbsp. coconut milk
- 8 tbsp. maple syrup for serving

Instructions:

Step 1: Preheat oven to 350 degrees F.

Step 2: Lay the coconut on a baking sheet in an even layer and toast for 4-5 minutes or until it begins to turn brown. Immediately transfer from hot pan to a blender jar.

Step 3: Add the baking powder, sea salt, almond flour, and lime to the blender and blend.

Step 4: Whisk the lime juice, eggs, honey, coconut milk, and water in a bowl until well combined. Add to the blender and blend on low until combined. The batter should be pourable, but not extremely thick. Add a tablespoon or two of water to thin out if necessary.

Step 5: Heat a griddle or cast-iron skillet to medium heat. Add the coconut oil and pour the batter into 3-inch pancakes. Cook until they are lightly brown on each side and ready to serve.

High Energy Breakfast Bars

Ingredients:

- 1 cup almonds
- 1 cup cashews
- ½ cup shredded coconut
- ¼ tsp. sea salt
- ¼ cup raw honey

Instructions:

Step 1: Put the almonds and cashews in a food processor and make sure to get them fully chopped up.

Step 2: Add the coconut and mix a little more, make sure not to over-chop. Move everything into a bowl and add the salt and honey. Mix thoroughly.

Step 3: Line a square baking sheet with parchment cooking paper. Press the mixture into the pan with your fingers and put the pan in the refrigerator. Chill for 2-3 hours until it becomes nice and firm.

Step 4: Cut it into snack sized energy bars.

Apple Cinnamon Muffins

Ingredients:

- 2 small diced apples
- 1 tbsp. lemon juice
- 5 large egg (cage free)
- ½ cup coconut flour
- 2 tbsp. cinnamon
- 1/8 tsp. ground nutmeg
- 1 tsp. baking soda
- 4 tbsp. coconut oil
- ¼ tsp. sea salt
- 1 package paper muffin liners

Instructions:

Step 1: Preheat over to 400 degrees F. Spray muffin tin with cooking spray or line with paper liners.

Step 2: Put the apples in a saucepan with the lemon juice and cover them. Add enough water to cover about half the saucepan.

Step 3: Bring the water to a boil and then reduce the heat for 10 minutes, until apples are broken down.

Step 4: Put everything into a blender and run until it become smooth. Let it cool for 5 minutes.

Step 5: When the apples get warm, add the remaining ingredients to the blender and blend until you have a nice thick batter.

Step 6: Pour the batter into your prepared muffin tin.

Step 7: Bake for roughly 15-20 minutes, until the muffins are lightly brown on top.

Mini Parsnip Cakes with Creamy Buffalo Dip

Ingredients:

- 6 medium parsnips about 1.5lbs
- 1 tsp. kosher salt
- 1 large egg (cage free)
- ½ tsp. garlic powder
- ½ tsp. onion powder
- 1 tbsp. coconut flour
- ½ tsp. freshly ground black pepper
- ¼ cup light olive oil
- ¼ cups Paleo mayo
- 2 tsp. hot pepper sauce

Instructions:

Step 1: Put all the parsnips in a saucepan and cover with cold water. Boil and cook them for 10 minutes and then let them cool off.

Step 2: When they have cooled off, shred the parsnips on a box grater and lay on paper towels. Sprinkle with the salt and let it sit for 5 minutes.

Step 3: Squeeze as much of the water out of the parsnips as you can and then put into a mixing bowl.

Step 4: Add the eggs, seasonings, and coconut flour and begin to mix everything thoroughly.

Step 5: Put the olive oil in a skillet and heat to medium heat. When the oil begins shimmering, scoop the parsnip mixture into the pan. Flatten the parsnips with a spatula and cook until golden brown on both sides.

Step 6: To serve, mix the mayo with the hot sauce and serve on the side of the cakes.

Blueberry Coconut Cereal

Ingredients:

- 2 cups chopped pecans
- 1/3 cups coconut oil
- 6 medium pitted dates
- 1 cup pumpkin seeds
- 1 tbsp. vanilla
- 2 tsp. cinnamon
- ½ tsp. sea salt
- ½ cup coconut flakes
- ½ cup blueberries

Instructions:

Step 1: Preheat oven to 325 degrees F.

Step 2: Put half of the pecans, coconut oil, and dates in a food processor or blender. Blend until it becomes finely ground.

Step 3: Add the remaining pecans and pumpkin seeds and blend again.

Step 4: Put all the blended food into a bowl and add the vanilla, cinnamon and salt. Stir it and spread it evenly on a baking sheet.

Step 5: Bake for about 25-30 minutes until it becomes lightly brown. After that let it cool and stir in the coconut and blueberries.

Step 6: Store in container until it's ready to serve.

Coconut Almond Pancakes

Ingredients:

- 1 medium ripe banana
- 1 cup coconut milk
- ¼ cup flax seeds
- 1 tbsp. coconut oil melted
- 1 cup almond meal
- 1 cup unsweetened coconut
- ½ cup orange juice
- 1 tsp. baking powder
- 1 tsp. cinnamon
- ¼ tsp. sea salt
- 1 cup fresh berries
- 4 tbsp. maple syrup

Instructions:

Step 1: Mash the banana in a large bowl and add the coconut milk, flax, and coconut oil. Let it sit for about 10-15 minutes.

Step 2: Add the remaining ingredients and mix well until you have a nice thick batter.

Step 3: Heat a skillet over medium heat and add a teaspoon of coconut oil. Drop the batter onto the skillet in small scoops and flatten slightly.

Step 4: Cook until the pancakes turn light brown on both sides and serve warm with fresh berries and some syrup.

Pumpkin Mango Smoothie

Ingredients:

- 1 medium frozen banana
- 1 medium mango
- 2 tbsp. coconut oil
- ½ cup organic pumpkin puree
- ½ tsp. cinnamon
- 1 cup almond milk
- 1 tbsp. collagen powder

Instructions:

- Put all the ingredients in a blender and blend until smooth and creamy. Serve immediately for a nice fresh taste.

Sweet Potato Breakfast Casserole

Ingredients:

The Casserole

- 2 medium sweet potatoes
- 2 cups unsweetened almond milk
- 1 cup coconut flakes
- 2 medium bananas
- 2 tbsp. of maple syrup
- 1 tbsp. vanilla
- 1 tsp. cinnamon
- ¼ tsp. sea salt

Toppings

- ½ cups chopped pecans
- 3 tbsp. melted coconut oil
- 1 tbsp. maple syrup
- 2 tbsp. almond flour

Instructions:

Step 1: Preheat oven to 375 degrees F.

Step 2: Boil a pot of water and add the sweet potatoes. Boil for 5-10 minutes until potatoes become lightly tender.

Step 3: Drain the sweet potatoes and set them aside

Step 4: Put the pot back to the stove and add the milk and coconut.

Step 5: Bring the water to a boil, turn the heat down to low and simmer them for 5-10 minutes.

Step 6: Turn of heat and add the sweet potatoes and bananas to the pot. Mash lightly and stir in the maple syrup, vanilla, cinnamon, and salt until it becomes well mixed.

Step 7: Put the mixture on a square baking pan or casserole dish.

Step 8: For the topping, mix the ingredients in a bowl until they are well mashed. Sprinkle the toping over the top of the casserole.

Step 9: Bake for 25-30 minutes, until top comes to a light brown color. Allow to cool slightly and serve warm.

Slow Cooker Paleo Breakfast Casserole

Ingredients:

- 1 sweet potato
- 8 eggs (cage free)
- ½-pound turkey bacon
- 1 chopped yellow onion
- 1 chopped red bell pepper
- (8 ounces) of mushrooms
- ½ packet taco seasoning
- Guacamole, salsa and jalapeno to garnish

Instructions:

Step 1: Fry the turkey bacon in a skillet until it gets crispy. Let it cool and then crumble it up into small pieces and then set it aside.

Step 2: Cook the onions in the same skillet until they are soft.

Step 3: Take the bacon, onions, sweet potato, bell pepper, mushrooms and eggs to the slow cooker. Stir to combine everything thoroughly.

Step 4: Put in your seasoning and stir it until it blends with the rest of the ingredients.

Step 5: Cook on low for 6-8 hours. Slice and serve with guacamole, salsa or jalapeno.

Paleo Lemon Poppyseed Muffins

Ingredients:

- 2 cups almond flour
- ¼ cup coconut flour
- ½ tsp. baking soda
- ½ tsp. baking powder
- ½ tsp. sea salt
- ½ cup unsweetened applesauce
- 2 lemons (about ½ cup)
- 3 large eggs (cage free)
- ¼ cup raw honey
- 1 tsp. vanilla extract
- 2 tbsp. poppy seeds

Instructions:

Step 1: Preheat oven to 350 degrees F.

Step 2: In a large bowl mix flour, coconut flour, baking soda, baking powder and sea salt.

Step 3: In another bowl mix applesauce, lemon juice, lemon zest, eggs, honey and vanilla extract.

Step 4: Add the wet ingredients to the dry ingredients and stir to combine.

Step 5: Stir in the poppy seeds

Step 6: Get a cooking tray and apply some cooking grease evenly along the tray.

Step 7: Bake for 25-30 minutes

Step 8: Remove them from the oven and let them cool for 5-10 minutes.

Hot Chocolate Pancakes with Salted Dulce de Leche

Ingredients:

For the pancakes:

- 1 cup almond meal
- 3 tbsp. coconut flour
- 3 tbsp. unsweetened cocoa powder
- ½ tsp. cinnamon
- 1/8 tsp. cayenne pepper
- 2 tsp. baking powder
- ¼ tsp. sea salt
- 1 cup unsweetened almond milk
- 2 eggs (cage free)
- 2 tbsp. maple syrup
- 1 tsp. vanilla extract

For the salted dulce de leche:

- ½ cup dates
- ¼ cup unsweetened almond milk
- 1 tsp. vanilla extract
- 1 tsp. melted coconut oil
- ¾ tsp. sea salt

Instructions:

For the Pancakes:

Step 1: In a large bowl mix the almond meal, coconut flour, cocoa powder, cinnamon, cayenne pepper, baking powder and sea salt thoroughly.

Step 2: In another bowl mix the almond milk, eggs, maple syrup and vanilla extract.

Step 3: Add the wet ingredients to the dry ingredients until they are well mixed. Let it sit for 5-10 minutes so the coconut flour absorbs the liquid.

Step 4: Heat a large cooking pan to medium heat and melt appropriately 1 teaspoon of coconut oil.

Step 5: Add 1/3 cup of batter per pancake and cook for 3 minutes or until all bubbles have aired out.

Step 6: Flip and cook for 1-2 more minutes.

For the salted dulce de leche:

Step 1: Strain dates and add them to a food processor or a blender.

Step 2: Add in all the other ingredients and blend them until they become well mixed.

Brussels Sprouts Breakfast Hash

Ingredients:

- 4 slices thick-cut bacon
- ½ red diced onion
- 1 sweet potato, peeled and cut into 1/2-inch cubes
- 2 minced garlic cloves
- 10-12 brussels sprouts, stems removed and sliced
- 3-4 large eggs (cage free)
- Salt and pepper

Instructions:

Step 1: Heat a skillet and add the four slices of bacon. Cook them until they are nice and crispy and remove over a paper towel.

Step 2: Reduce the heat under the skillet and add onion and the sweet potato. Cook them until the sweet potato has softened, about 5-10 minutes, then stir in the garlic and cook for about another minute.

Step 3: Add sliced brussels sprouts and stir to mix with everything. Cook them until they are nice and soft.

Step 4: At the same time poach or fry eggs, cook them until they are done.

CHAPTER 6

PALEO LUNCH RECIPES

Paleo Banana Pancakes

Ingredients:

- 1 ¼ cup almond flour
- ¼ cup coconut flour
- ½ tsp. baking soda
- ¼ tsp. sea salt
- 1 cup coconut milk
- 1 ripe banana
- 3 large eggs (cage free)
- 1 tsp. vanilla extract
- 1 tbsp. raw honey (optional)

Instructions:

Step 1: Sift and mix the dry ingredients.

Step 2: In a medium sized bowl, whisk together the coconut milk, banana, eggs and vanilla.

Step 3: Add the dry ingredients to the wet ingredients and whisk until they are well mixed together.

Step 4: Preheat a pan on a medium heat and oil it up with a layer of coconut oil.

Step 5: Pour out two tablespoons of batter onto the pan to make the pancakes.

Step 6: Cook the pancakes for 2-3 minutes per side or until they get golden brown on the top.

Sausage Broccoli Egg Muffins

Ingredients:

- 9 large eggs (cage free)
- 8 ounces ground sausage (cooked)
- 1 cup chopped steamed broccoli
- ¼ tsp. sea salt
- ¼ tsp. pepper

Instructions:

Step 1: Preheat oven to 350 degrees F.

Step 2: Grease a muffin tin with coconut oil and set aside.

Step 3: Whisk together the eggs in a mixing bowl and add in the ground sausage, broccoli, salt and pepper.

Step 4: Pour the mixture into the muffin tins and bake for 25-30 minutes or until the eggs have set.

Eggs Benedict with Avocado Sauce

Ingredients:

- 5 strips of bacon
- 4 eggs (cage free)
- Sea salt and freshly ground black pepper

Ingredients for the avocado sauce

- 1 medium avocado
- ¼ cup lemon juice
- ½ tsp. garlic powder
- 1/3 cup olive oil or water

Eggs benedict Prep:

Instructions:

Step 1: Preheat oven to 400 degrees F.

Step 2: On a cooking sheet, put the bacon into four separate bases for the eggs. Cook the bacon bases in the oven for 15 to 20 minutes.

Step 3: Puree the avocado, lemon juice and garlic powder in a food processor or blender until it gets nice and smooth.

Step 4: Add the olive oil or water until you get a thick but pourable consistency. Season to taste with sea salt.

Step 5: Boil a pot of water and drop the eggs in it and let them cook until the whites are set (2 to 5 minutes). Remove and repeat for the rest of the eggs.

Step 6: Divide the bacon evenly among the plates, top with the peached eggs and pour the avocado sauce on top of each egg.

Paleo Coffee Cake Banana Bread

Ingredients:

- 3 brown bananas
- ¼ cup maple syrup
- 1 tsp. vanilla extract
- 3 eggs (cage free)
- ½ cup almond butter
- ¼ cup coconut flour
- ½ tsp. baking soda
- ½ tsp. baking powder
- 1 tsp. cinnamon

*** add a pinch of salt ***

For the toppings:

- 4 tbsp. grass fed butter or coconut oil
- 2 tbsp. coconut sugar
- 2 tbsp. almond flour
- 1 tsp. cinnamon
- ¼ cup crushed pecans

Instructions:

Step 1: Preheat oven to 350 degrees F.

Step 2: Grease a baking dish with oil then line the middle with parchment paper.

Step 3: In a large bowl, mix together the bananas, maple syrup, vanilla extract, eggs, and almond butter.

Step 4: Add in the coconut flour, baking soda, baking powder, cinnamon and salt and mix it thoroughly.

Step 5: Pour the batter into a baking dish.

Step 6: In a small bowl, add butter, coconut sugar, almond flour, cinnamon, and pecans. Mix the toppings together thoroughly.

Step 7: Sprinkle the toppings on top of the banana bread mixture.

Step 8: Place the bread dish on a baking sheet and bake for 45-50 minutes.

Step 9: Take it out of the oven and place on cooling rack and let it rest for 5-10 minutes before cutting up and serving.

Lettuce Tacos with Chipotle Chicken

Ingredients:

- 400 g of boneless chicken breast cut into thin strips
- 1 red sliced onion
- 400 g of chopped tomatoes
- 1 tbsp. of finely chopped chipotle in adobo sauce
- ½ tsp. cumin
- Pinch of brown sugar and salt and pepper for seasoning
- Lettuce leaves for the tacos
- Fresh coriander leaves
- Pickled jalapeno chilies
- Slices of avocado or make some guacamole
- Fresh tomatoes and slices of spring onion to make rustic salsa
- Lime wedges for zest

Instructions:

Step 1: Heat the olive oil in a frying pan and fry your chicken pieces until they turn golden. After they are done set them aside.

Step 2: In the same pan, add some more olive oil and frying your onion until it gets soft.

Step 3: Add your tomatoes, cumin, sugar and chipotle and simmer for around 15-25 minutes until the tomato sauce starts to thicken.

Step 4: Put the chicken back into the sauce and cook for about 5-10 minutes.

Step 5: Take all the other ingredients to make your tacos in separate bowls and serve so you can make your own.

Cuban Picadillo Lettuce Wraps

Ingredients:

For the Picadillo:

- 1-pound grass fed ground beef
- 2 tbsp. coconut oil
- 1 medium diced onion
- 1 large green bell pepper
- ½ tsp. salt
- 1 tsp. black pepper
- 1 tsp. ground cumin
- ½ tsp. ground cinnamon
- 1 14 oz can whole tomatoes
- ¼ cup currants
- 2 tbsp. green olives with pimiento
- 2 tbsp. drained capers
- 2 tbsp. olive brine

For the Pico de Gallo

- 1/3 cup minced shallot or red onion
- 2/3 cup diced tomatoes
- 2 tbsp. minced cilantro
- 2 tbsp. fresh lime juice

** sprinkle some salt **

To Serve (optional)

- Lettuce leaves or cabbages leaves
- Cooked brown or white rice
- Chopped cilantro

Instructions:

Step 1: Heat a large pan or oven over medium heat with some olive oil.

Step 2: Add beef and crumble it and stir as it cooks. Let it cook slowly and set it aside.

Step 3: Add some olive oil to a pan. Add the onions and cook them until they begin to soften, for roughly 5 minutes. Add the bell pepper and cook a few more minutes. Add in the garlic, salt, black pepper, cumin, and cinnamon and stir for about a minute until they fully blend together.

Step 4: Add cooked beef, canned tomatoes, currants, diced olives, capers, and olive brine. Break up tomatoes into small pieces while the mixture comes to a boil.

Step 5: Reduce the heat to low temp and cover the food and let it simmer for 10-25 minutes.

Step 6: Prep the Pico De Gallo. Mix the chopped shallot, tomatoes, cilantro, lime juice, and salt.

Step 7: Fill the lettuce leaves with beef mixture and enjoy any way you see fit.

California Turkey and Bacon Lettuce Wraps with Basil-Mayo

Ingredients:

- 1 head iceberg lettuce
- 4 slices deli turkey (gluten free)
- 4 slices of bacon (gluten free)
- 1 avocado
- 1 roma tomato

For the Basil-Mayo:

- 1/2 cup mayonnaise (gluten free)
- 6 large basil leaves
- 1 tsp. lemon juice
- 1 garlic clove
- Pinch of salt and pepper

Instructions:

For the Basil-Mayo:

Step 1: Mix the ingredients in a food processor or blender and make sure they become smooth. Chop the basil and garlic then mix all ingredients together.

Step 2: Lay out the lettuce leaves then layer on one slice of turkey and slather with Basil-Mayo. Put on a second slice of turkey followed by bacon, and a few slices of both avocado and tomato.

Step 3: Season with salt and pepper then fold the bottom up, tuck the sides in, and roll like a burrito.

Steak & Sriracha Lettuce Wraps

Ingredients:

- 1 pound of fajita strips
- 1 large diced onion
- 3 cloves of diced garlic
- 1 diced bell pepper
- Pea shots
- 2 tbsp. sriracha sauce
- 2 tsp. coconut
- 1 tbsp. sesame oil
- Green onions
- Romaine lettuce

Instructions:

Step 1: In a medium sized pan add some olive oil and heat thoroughly.

Step 2: Add the fajita meat and cook for about 5 minutes.

Step 3: Add the onions and bell peppers and continue to cook until they get nice and brown.

Step 4: Add the garlic, sesame oil, sriracha sauce, coconut and pea shots.

Step 5: After the meat and veggies have absorbed the sauce, turn the heat down on low and begin to serve them on the lettuce wraps.

Cajun Garlic Shrimp Noodle Bowls

Ingredients:

- 3 crushed cloves of garlic
- 3 tbsp. of butter (grass fed)
- 15-30 jumbo shrimp
- Pinch of Cajun seasoning
- Dash of cayenne
- ½ tsp. seal salt
- 1 tsp. paprika
- Red pepper flakes
- 1 tsp. garlic granules
- 1 tsp. of onion powder

(Optional extras)

- 2 zucchinis (diced)
- Red peppers (diced)
- 1 onion, sliced (diced)
- Butter

Instructions:

Step 1: Chop up your zucchini and mix with your Cajun seasoning and shrimp in a bowl.

Step 2: Melt butter and garlic in a large sized pan.

Step 3: Add in red pepper and onion and sauté for 5-10 minutes.

Step 4: Add in the shrimp and let it cook until it mixes and cooks nicely.

Step 5: In another pan heat up the remaining tablespoon of butter and add zucchini for 5-10 minutes.

Step 6: Put your zucchini noodles in a bowl and add the Cajun shrimp and veggies on top.

Paleo Egg Roll In A Bowl

Ingredients:

- 1 head of chopped cabbage
- 2 large carrots
- 1 tbsp. coconut oil
- ½ cup coconut aminos
- 1 tbsp. sesame oil
- 2 minced garlic cloves
- 4 diced green onions

Instructions:

Step 1: Melt the coconut oil in a pan on medium heat.

Step 2: Add the carrots and the cabbage.

Step 3: Sautee the carrots and the cabbage until they get soft. Add a little water if they get too dry.

Step 4: Add the sesame oil and the ½ cup of coconut aminos.

Step 5: Add the garlic and cook until the flavors are well blended. After they are well blended add the green onions.

Mexican Paleo Super Food Bowls

Ingredients:

For the French fries:

- 3 large carrots
- 1 sweet potato
- 1 tbsp. of taco seasoning
- Pinch of salt
- A drizzle of olive oil

For the chicken:

- 1 chicken breast (cage free) (cut into small pieces)
- 2 tbsp. ketchup (organic)
- 1 tbsp. of raw honey
- 1 tbsp. of taco seasoning
- Pinch of salt

For the Pico de Gallo:

- 3 large diced roma tomatoes
- 1 large diced red onion
- Shredded cilantro
- Lime juice
- 1 chopped jalapeno pepper
- Pinch of salt and pepper

(Optional extras)

- 1 mashed avocado
- Spinach
- Fried eggs

Instructions:

Step 1: Preheat oven to 450 degrees F.

Step 2: Cut the carrots and sweet potatoes into bite sized fries. Season with taco seasoning and put them on a baking tray.

Step 3: Drizzle them with olive oil and bake them for 20-25 minutes.

Step 4: Heat up some olive oil in a pan and add chicken pieces and cook until they become golden brown. Sprinkle taco seasoning, ketchup and some honey until the flavors blend with the chicken pieces.

Step 5: Slice tomatoes, onions and jalapenos. Toss them in a bowl with the lime juice and the chopped cilantro and mix them well. Add some eggs to the mix if you desire.

Bowl of Doom

Ingredients:

- 3 sweet potatoes
- 1 pound of ground beef
- 5 green onions
- 1 avocado
- 2-4 eggs (cage free)

For the Salsa:

- 1 tbsp. ground cumin
- Pinch of salt and pepper
- 1 tbsp. olive oil
- 1 tbsp. coconut oil

Instructions:

Step 1: Peel the sweet potatoes and then cut them up into small pieces. Smaller pieces will cook faster.

Step 2: Once you have cut the potatoes up, heat up a pan on medium heat with some olive oil.

Step 3: Add the sweet potatoes once the olive oil comes to a nice simmer and then add the coconut oil, salt and pepper to help soften them up some more and bring in additional flavor.

Step 4: Move the cooked potatoes into a separate bowl and then use the leftover oil to cook your ground beef. Season the beef with 1 tablespoon of ground cumin, 2 teaspoons of salt and 2 teaspoons of the garlic powder.

Step 5: Chop up the green onions and heat up a separate pan to cook your eggs in.

Step 6: Once the beef begins to turn brown, add the green onions to the mix and cook for a couple more minutes until the flavors have blended together. After the flavors have blended, add in your sliced up sweet potatoes. Cook and mix everything thoroughly.

Step 7: Cook 2-4 eggs in the separate pan or however you like. Make sure to cook them in olive oil with a pinch of salt and cracked pepper. Then cut up the avocado in half and slice it down into small pieces.

Step 8: Put some salsa in a separate bowl and prep your bowl of doom however you want.

Burrito Bowl Date Night Recipe

Ingredients:

- 2 cloves of garlic
- ¼ cup olive oil
- 1 tbsp. chili powder
- 1 tbsp. apple cider vinegar
- 1 tbsp. of lime juice
- 2 tsp. of sea salt
- 1 tsp. black pepper
- 1 tsp. of paprika
- ½ tsp. dried oregano
- 2-4 pounds of boneless chicken thighs or breasts

For the Pico De Gallo:

- 1 large tomato
- ½ tsp. sea salt
- ½ diced small onion
- ¼ cup chopped cilantro
- 1 tbsp. of lime juice

For the Cilantro Rice:

- 2 cups of steamed rice
- 2 tsp. of avocado oil
- 1 tbsp. of lime juice
- 1 tsp. lemon juice
- ½ tsp. of sea salt
- ½ cup cilantro

To Serve:

- 1 shredded head of romaine lettuce
- 1 batch of guacamole
- 1 cup of sour cream
- 1 cup of cheese

Instructions:

Step 1: Blend olive oil, garlic, chili powder, lime juice, vinegar, salt, pepper, paprika and oregano in a blender or food processor until they have mixed well.

Step 2: Take a small Ziplog bag and put the chicken in there to marinate with the sauce for 6-8 hours.

Step 3: Mix all the listed ingredients for the Pico de Gallo.

Step 4: Take a skillet or cooking pan or even fire up your grill and cook the chicken until it becomes about halfway done. After you cook it about halfway, take it off and cut it into small pieces. After you cut it into small pieces, continue to cook it until it becomes ready.

Step 5: Place the steamed rice in a medium sized bowl and mix in the avocado oil. Add the lime, lemon juice and salt and stir everything until the flavors have been blended together. Add in the cilantro and see how everything tastes. Add in more flavors as you see fit to your liking.

Step 6: Serve the burrito bowls with as much rice, chicken and guacamole as you want.

Cuban Sandwich Bowls

Ingredients:

- 1-pound pork tenderloin
- 1 tbsp. apple cider vinegar
- ½ cup applesauce

For the Plantain Chips:

- 2 green plantains
- 1 tsp. garlic powder
- 1 cup of water
- 3 minced garlic cloves
- 5 tbsp. of coconut oil
- Pinch of salt

For the mojo sauce:

- 1 tbsp. olive oil
- 3 minced garlic cloves
- 1/3 cup orange juice
- Juice of 2 small limes
- 1/8 tsp. ground cumin
- ½ tsp. salt
- ¼ tsp. cracked pepper

(Optional Toppings)

- ½ pound of ham
- 6 cups of shredded cabbage
- Salt and vinegar chips
- 1 avocado
- Mustard

Instructions:

Step 1: Put the pork in a slow cooker and pour applesauce and apple cider vinegar all over it. Set to high and cook for 6 hours. When it is done cooking shred and toss it with ½ cup of mojo sauce.

For the Mojo Sauce:

Step 1: In a medium sized pan heat up 1 tablespoon of olive oil. Put the 3 garlic cloves in there until they turn light brown for about 1-2 minutes.

Step 2: Put the garlic in a small bowl and mix in the remaining olive oil, orange juice, lime juice, cumin, salt, and pepper.

For the Plantain Chips:

Step 1: Pour one cup of water, 1 teaspoon garlic powder, and 3 minced garlic cloves in a medium sized bowl.

Step 2: Peel the plantains and cut them into small slices.

Step 3: Heat up the coconut oil in a large sized pan. Fry the plantains for 1-2 minutes per side until they become light brown.

Step 4: Mash the plantains until they are down to about half their original size. Soak in the garlic water for 1-2 minutes, and fry once more for about 1-minute per side. This will help them absorb a ton of flavor.

Step 5: Move them to a new plate and season lightly with some salt.

Step 6: In a large bowl, put in 2 cups of cabbage or lettuce. Mix it in with pork, avocado, pickles, plantain chips, and as much mustard as you see fit. Put the mojo sauce on the side.

BLT Bowl (my favorite)

Ingredients:

- 1 avocado
- 2 tomatoes
- 2 romaine lettuce hearts
- 1 cucumber
- ½ cup chopped cilantro
- 5 pieces of bacon
- ½ cup of feta cheese

Instructions:

Step 1: Cook the bacon until it comes to a nice even crisp.

Step 2: While the bacon cooks, chop the remaining ingredients down into bite sized pieces.

Step 3: Mix everything into a bowl, followed by the bacon once it is done cooking. Crumble your feta cheese over the top of your bowl.

Step 4: Pour 2 shot glasses of olive oil into a cup. Add balsamic vinegar, one teaspoon of mustard, the juice from the small lemon and a pinch of salt.

Put this sauce over your bowl.

Healthy Taco Salad

Ingredients:

- 1 tbsp. olive oil
- 8 oz. chicken breast cut into bite-sized pieces
- 2 cups sliced carrots
- 1 red bell pepper
- ½ cup chopped white onion
- 2 tsp. minced garlic
- 2 tsp. ground cumin
- Pinch of sea salt
- 1 avocado
- 1 lime (juiced)
- 1 cup salsa
- 2 cups of chopped tomatoes
- ½ cup chopped cucumber
- ½ chopped cilantro
- Spinach
- 2 wide-mouth sized mason jars

Instructions:

Step 1: Heat up ½ tablespoon of olive oil in a large pan.

Step 2: Cook the chicken until it begins to turn golden brown. Once it has cooked thoroughly, set it aside in a medium sized bowl.

Step 3: Add the remaining ½ tablespoon of olive oil into the pan and turn to medium heat.

Step 4: Cook the carrots until they start to get soft, for about 5 minutes. Turn the heat down to low and add in the onion, pepper and garlic.

Step 5: While the vegetables cook, put the cumin seeds in a dry pan over high heat and toast them for about 2 minutes until they turn golden.

Step 6: Move them to a cutting board and crush them up. Add the crushed seeds into the pant with the veggies and season with sea salt. Mix everything thoroughly until the flavors have blended.

Step 7: Put the avocado and the lime juice into a food processor or blender and blend until it turns creamy.

Step 8: Place ½ cup of salsa in the bottom of each mason jar and spread it out evenly. Divide the avocado and lime mixture on top and gently spread it out.

Step 9: Split the roasted veggies and add the chicken. Pack everything in tightly.

Step 10: After you have added the chicken, place the tomatoes in, followed by the cucumbers. Finish off by adding the cilantro and spinach.

Store in the refrigerator to lock in the fresh flavors.

Grilled Paleo Pizza

Ingredients:

For the Crust:

- ¼ cup of coconut flour
- 1 cup tapioca starch
- 2 eggs
- 1 cup of water
- Pinch of salt

For the Toppings:

- Your favorite pasta sauce or pizza sauce
- Tomatoes
- Jalapeno peppers
- Watercress or spinach
- Chopped onions
- Chopped peppers
- Fresh Basil

Instructions:

Step 1: Mix the ingredients together for the crust until smooth.

Step 2: Preheat your cooking pan or grill.

Step 3: Heat a large pan over high heat until it gets hot. Pour in a little bit of olive oil to grease the pan and get it ready for cooking.

Step 4: Pour in half of the crust mixture and cook it until the top begins to bubble.

Step 5: Cook until it begins to get crispy. After it cooks move it to a plate and top with the toppings from our list.

Step 6: Move the pizzas to the grill and let them cook for about 5-10 minutes or until the crust is golden brown.

Paleo Salmon Salad Power Bowls (my second favorite)

Ingredients:

- 6-oz ounce baked salmon
- 4-5 cups of seasonal greens
- ½ cup sliced zucchini and squash
- ½ cup of raspberries
- 1 tbsp. balsamic vinegar
- 2 tbsp. olive oil
- Pinch of sea salt
- Pinch of black pepper
- 2 thyme springs
- Lemon juice

Instructions:

Step 1: Slice your zucchini and squash and mix it a pan with ½ tbsp. olive oil and add little bit of pepper/salt.

Step 2: Preheat oven to 400 degrees F.

Step 3: Drizzle 1 tbsp. of olive oil, lemon, pepper and a pinch of salt and cook your salmon for about 10-15 minutes.

Step 4: After the zucchini and the salmon are cooked, build your bowl any way you see fit with the provided ingredients.

Add raspberries last with some lemon juice on top and drizzle some parmesan.

Enjoy!

Antipasto Salad Recipe

Ingredients:

- 1 large chopped head of romaine
- 4 ounces prosciutto
- 4 ounces of salami
- ½ cup sliced artichoke hearts
- ½ cup of mixed olives
- ½ cup picked sweet peppers
- Italian dressing

Instructions:

Step 1: Mix all the ingredients in a large serving bowl.

Step 2: Toss in as much Italian dressing as you want

CHAPTER 7

PALEO DINNER RECIPES

Paleo Avocado Tuna Salad

Ingredients:

- 1 avocado
- 1 juiced lemon
- 1 tbsp. chopped onion
- 5 ounces of wild tuna
- Pinche of sea salt
- Ground pepper

Instructions:

Step 1: Cut up the avocado in half and put into a bowl, leaving the shell of avocado flesh out.

Step 2: Add onions and lemon juice to the avocado in the bowl and mash them together. Add tuna, salt and pepper and mix to combine.

Step 3: Fill the avocado shells with tuna salad and enjoy.

Simple and yummy!

Thai Chopped Chicken Salad with Chili Vinaigrette

Ingredients:

- 1 large chopped head of romaine lettuce
- 2 grilled chicken breasts seasoned
- 1 tsp. oregano
- 1 tsp. garlic granules
- Pinch of sea salt
- ½ cup broccoli
- 1 tbsp. chili paste

Mango and Cabbage Slaw:

- ½ cup sliced mango
- ½ cup chopped cabbage
- 1 tsp. apple cider vinegar

Roasted Red Peppers & Tomatoes:

- ½ cup chopped roasted red peppers
- ½ cup chopped grape tomatoes
- 1 tbsp. Chili vinaigrette
- 2 tbsp. rice vinegar
- 1 tsp. coconut aminos
- 1 tbsp. extra-virgin olive oil
- 1 tsp. fresh lime juice
- 1 tsp. chili paste
- ½ tsp. freshly grated ginger

Instructions:

Step 1: Cook or grill chicken on your grill pan or BBQ.

Step 2: Sauté the broccoli until it gets soft.

Step 3: In a separate bowl mix the mango and cabbage with 1 tsp. of apple cider vinegar.

Step 4: Chop the tomatoes, lettuce and roasted red peppers.

Step 5: Mix everything together and serve.

Rosemary Lamb Burgers with Pesto Sauce

Ingredients:

- 1 pound of ground lamb
- 1 tsp. sea salt
- 1 tbs. of fresh rosemary
- 1 tbs. coconut oil

For the Pesto:

- 1 bunch of fresh basil leaves
- ½ cup of olive oil
- 1 tsp. of fresh lemon juice
- 1 chopped clove of garlic
- ¼ tsp. sea salt
- 1 chopped clove of garlic
- ¼ tsp. sea salt
- 1/3 cup hemp seeds

For the Garnish:

- Salad greens of your choice
- Olive oil
- White wine vinegar
- Pinch of salt and pepper

Instructions:

Step 1: Mix the ground lamb, rosemary, and salt until they are well combined and form them into 1-inch thick patties.

Step 2: Melt fat or heat up oil of choice in pan over medium heat. Cook the patties until their sides turn brown.

Step 3: At the same time, place the basil, olive oil, lemon, garlic, and salt into a food processor or blender and blend everything thoroughly.

Step 4: Add the hemp seeds and mix until desired pesto gets creamy. Feel free to add a pinch of salt and pepper.

Step 5: Mix your choice of greens in some olive oil, white wine vinegar with a pinch of salt and pepper. Put your lamb burger on top of your greens or enjoy on the side. Add some pesto sauce on your burger and enjoy!

Honey and Sesame-Glazed Chicken Breasts with Green Beans

Ingredients:

- 6 tbsp. of chicken stock
- ½ cup honey
- 2 tbsp. sesame oil
- 1 ½ tbsp. mustard
- 4 boneless chicken breasts
- ¾ tsp. sea salt
- ½ tsp. freshly ground black pepper
- 2 tsp. sesame seeds
- 2 green beans (8-ounce)
- 1 tbsp. unsalted butter
- 2 tbsp. almonds

Instructions:

Step 1: Combine the chicken stock, 1/3 cup of honey, 1 tablespoon of sesame oil, and mustard in a medium sized pan and let it simmer and mix for about 10 minutes.

Step 2: Heat a large pan skillet over medium heat with a splay of sesame oil.

Step 3: Season the chicken breasts with ½ teaspoon of salt and ¼ teaspoon of pepper.

Step 4: Add the chicken to the pan and cook for 7 minutes on each side or until it looks done. Drizzle honey over the chicken and sprinkle sesame seeds over it.

Step 5: Make the green beans according to the directions on the package. Mix the green beans with ¼ teaspoon of salt, ¼ teaspoon of pepper, and butter. Add some almonds if desired.

Beef and Broccoli Stuffed Sweet Potatoes

Ingredients:

- 4 sweet potatoes
- 1 tbsp. olive oil
- 1 cup chopped red onion
- ¾ cup chopped red bell peppers
- 4 minced garlic cloves
- 2 tsp. chili powder
- ½ tsp. sea salt
- ½ tsp. ground cumin
- ¼ tsp. ground red pepper
- 12 ounces of top sirloin
- 2 cups frozen broccoli florets
- ¼ cup green onions

Instructions:

Step 1: Oil up the sweet potatoes with 1 ½ teaspoons of olive oil.

Step 2: Put them in the microwave on high for 12 to 15 minutes or until potatoes become tender and steamy.

Step 3: Heat a large pan over medium heat with a splash of olive oil. Make sure to cover the pan thoroughly with oil.

Step 4: Add the onions and red bell peppers and cook for 5-10 minutes or until they begin to get tender.

Step 5: Mix in the garlic and stir thoroughly. Stir in the chili powder, ¼ teaspoon of salt, red pepper and ground cumin.

Step 6: Add the beef and cook for about 5-10 minutes or until it beings to turn brown.

Step 7: Make the broccoli according to the directions of the package and add it into the rest of the beef mixture. Cut up the potatoes lengthwise.

Step 8: Top the potatoes evenly with the beef mixture and add the remaining ¼ teaspoon of salt and green onions.

Creamy Sweet Potato Soup

Ingredients:

- 2 pounds of sweet potatoes
- ¼ cup of water
- 2 tsp. of olive oil
- 1 cup chopped onion
- ½ tsp. ground cumin
- ¼ tsp. red pepper
- 4 cups chicken stock
- ¼ tsp. salt
- 6 bacon slices
- 1-ounce parmesan cheese
- 2 tbsp. parsley leaves

Instructions:

Step 1: Add ¼ cup of water into a baking dish and add the cut-up potatoes in it. Microwave on high for roughly 15 minutes or until the potatoes tender up.

Step 2: Heat up the cooking pan on medium heat and add olive oil and cover up the pan. Add in 1 cup of the chopped onion until it comes to a light simmer. Shortly after, add in ½ teaspoon of ground cumin and ¼ teaspoon red pepper.

Step 3: Add the chicken stock to the cooking pan and bring it to a nice boil.

Step 4: Put half of the sweet potatoes and half of stock mixture in a blender or food processor and blend until it becomes smooth.

Step 5: Pour the soup into a large bowl. Repeat procedure with remaining sweet potato and stock mixture. Stir in a pinch of salt and pepper. Divide the soup evenly amount 4-6 bowls, add in the cooked bacon slices and sprinkle parmesan cheese over the top. Add some parsley for additional flavor if desired.

Blackened Streak Salad

Ingredients:

- ½ tsp. sea salt
- ½ tsp. black pepper
- ½ tsp. paprika
- ¼ tsp. garlic powder
- 1 flank steak (12 oz)
- ¼ cup olive oil
- 2 tbsp. balsamic vinegar
- 1 tsp. mustard
- 4 cups arugula
- ½ cup red onion
- ½ avocado

Instructions:

Step 1: Heat a grill pan over medium temperature.

Step 2: In a separate bowl mix salt, pepper, paprika, and garlic powder together and cover the flank steak evenly.

Step 3: Add the flank steak to the pan and grill 5-7 minutes on each side or until its fully cooked to your liking.

Step 4: Put the flank steak on a cutting board and cut it up into small slices.

Step 5: Mix together olive oil, vinegar, and mustard in a medium-sized blow and stir it until it blends together nicely.

Step 6: Add the steak, arugula, and onion and mix it together. Top it off with some avocado and serve warm.

Skillet Chicken with Escarole and Pecorino

Ingredients:

- 1 pound of escarole, cut into medium sized pieces
- 2 tsp. olive oil
- 4 chicken breasts (4-ounces each)
- ½ tsp. sea salt
- ¼ tsp. ground black pepper
- 4 garlic cloves
- ¼ teaspoon crushed red pepper
- ½ red onion
- 2 tsp. fish sauce
- ¼ cup sliced carrots
- ½ ounce shaved pecorino cheese

Instructions:

Step 1: Boil a saucepan of water on high heat.

Step 2: Add escarole and cook for 2-5 minutes. After it is done cooking drain it.

Step 3: Heat up 2 teaspoons of olive oil in a medium sized pan. Lay out the chicken and season with salt and pepper evenly. Cook the chicken for 5 minutes on each side or until done. Move it to a serving plate.

Step 4: Turn down the heat. Add 2 tablespoons of olive oil and garlic and cook for 1-3 minutes. Add in red pepper and onion and cook 1-3 minutes.

Step 5: Take out the garlic from the pan and add the escarole and cook for 1-3 minutes. After that stir in fish sauce.

Eat and Enjoy!

Paleo Spaghetti Squash Shakshuka

Ingredients:

- 1 spaghetti squash
- 2 tbsp. olive oil
- ½ yellow onion
- 1 large chopped garlic clove
- 1 minced red pepper
- 1 chopped jalapeno
- Unsalted tomatoes
- 1 tsp. cumin
- ¾ tsp. chili powder
- ½ tsp. kosher salt
- 2 large eggs (cage free)
- 2 tbsp. chopped cilantro

Instructions:

Step 1: Preheat oven to 425 degrees F.

Step 2: Take a fork and poke the spaghetti squash several times all over so it creates holes for it to breathe out of.

Step 3: Microwave for 7-10 minutes on high. Cut squash in half and take out the seeds.

Step 4: In a medium-sized pan on medium heat, add olive oil, onion, and peppers. Cook until slightly softened for about 5-7 minutes.

Step 5: Add the garlic and sauté for 1-3 minutes. Add the canned tomatoes, cumin, chili powder, salt and pepper, and let them simmer for 10 minutes until the flavors have blended.

Step 6: To make the dish, split up the sauce among each of the 4 squash halves. Use a spoon or spatula and mix the tomato sauce with squash strands. Make a scoop in the center of each squash and crack an egg into the middle.

Step 7: Place each squash half on a baking sheet. Use some aluminum foil to secure the squash halves if they start to roll. Bake for 10-15 minutes.

Step 8: After they are done baking remove them from the oven, top with cilantro, and serve immediately.

Shrimp Cauliflower Fried Rice

Ingredients:

- ½ pound peeled shrimp
- 1 tsp. grated ginger
- ¼ tsp. crushed red pepper
- 2 tsp. sesame oil
- ½ cup chopped red bell pepper
- ½ cup sliced green onions
- 1 tbsp. minced garlic
- 4 cups of diced cauliflower
- 1 large egg (cage free)
- 1 tbsp. water

Instructions:

Step 1: Put the shrimp, ginger, and crushed red pepper in a medium sized bowl.

Step 2: Heat up the sesame oil in a large nonstick pan over high heat.

Step 3: Add the bell pepper, green onions, and garlic and stir-fry them for 1 to 2 minutes or until they get tender.

Step 4: Add the shrimp mixture to the pan and stir-fry them for 4 to 5 minutes or until the shrimp are done. Add the diced cauliflower and stir-fry for 2 minutes or until it cooks well.

Step 5: Move the rice mixture to the sides of the pan, forming a well in the center. Add the egg to the center of the pan and cook it for about 1 minute.

Step 6: Mix it in with the rice mixture and stir-fry it until the egg gets fully cooked. Add in the water and cook until everything blends well together (another 5 minutes).

Paleo Seared Scallops with Cauliflower Puree

Ingredients:

- 2 cups chopped cauliflower
- 1 cup peeled potato
- 1 cup water
- ½ cup chicken broth
- 1 tbsp. olive oil
- 1 ½ pounds of sea scallops
- ¾ tsp. sea salt
- ½ tsp. ground black pepper
- 1 ½ tbsp. ghee
- 1/8 tsp. crushed red pepper

Instructions:

Step 1: Pour ½ cup chicken broth, 1 cup of water, 1 cup peeled potato and 2 cups chopped cauliflower in the saucepan and bring it to a nice boil. Cook and stir until they have cooked nicely.

Step 2: Heat a large pan over high heat and drizzle olive oil over the pan.

Step 3: Pat scallops dry with some paper towels and add with ¼ teaspoon salt and black pepper.

Step 4: Add the scallops to a cooking pan and cook them for 2-3 minutes on each side. Once the scallops are done cooking remove them from the pan.

Step 5: Put the cauliflower mixture in a blender or food processor. Add ½ teaspoon of salt, ghee, and red pepper. Blend the ingredients until it becomes like a puree. Serve it with the scallops and enjoy

Roasted Shrimp and Broccoli

Ingredients:

- 5 cups of broccoli florets
- 1 tbsp. grated lemon
- 1 tbsp. lemon juice
- ½ tsp. sea salt
- ½ tsp. ground black pepper
- 1 ½ pounds peeled shrimp
- 2 tbsp. olive oil
- ¼ tsp. crushed red pepper

Instructions:

Step 1: Preheat oven to 425 F.

Step 2: Boil the broccoli in some water until it becomes soft. After it is done boiling put it in a small bowl.

Step 3: Mix the lemon juice, ¼ teaspoon of sea salt, and ¼ teaspoon black pepper in a medium sized bowl.

Step 4: Add the shrimp to the bowl and toss it until the flavors mix well. Put the shrimp and broccoli on a cooking pan coated with some olive oil or cooking spray.

Step 5: Bake at 425 F for 8-10 minutes or until the shrimp are thoroughly cooked.

Enjoy!

Paleo Skillet Chicken with Seared Avocados

Ingredients:

- 1 tbsp. olive oil
- 4 boneless chicken breasts (6-ounce each)
- ½ tsp. sea salt
- ½ tsp. black pepper
- ½ tsp. ground chili powder
- 2 small avocados (pitted and split in half)
- ¼ tsp. coconut sugar
- 2 peeled and chopped red onions
- 4 chopped green onions
- 1 poblano pepper
- 3 tbsp. fresh lime juice
- 1 tbsp. liquid aminos
- 8 cilantro sprigs
- 4 lime wedges

Instructions:

Step 1: Preheat oven to 425 degrees F.

Step 2: Heat a large pan skillet over medium heat and drizzle some oil to a pan and coat it evenly.

Step 3: Season the chicken breasts with ¼ teaspoon salt, black pepper, and chili powder.

Step 4: Add the chicken breast to the cooking pan and cook for 2-3 minutes per side or until golden brown. Move the chicken from the pan, it will not be fully cooked yet.

Step 5: Clean the pan off and season the avocados with coconut sugar and cook them in the pan for no more than 2 minutes. After they are done cooking remove them from the pan.

Step 6: Add the red onions and cook them for 3 minutes or until charred. Add green onions and poblano and cook for 3 more minutes.

Step 7: Separate the red onions into rings and add them to the green onions and poblano. Add in the lime juice and liquid aminos.

Step 8: Put the chicken and avocados into the onion mixture. Place a cooking pan in the oven and bake at 425 degrees F for 7-10 minutes or until the chicken is done.

Step 9: Take the cooking pan out of the oven and garnish your dish with cilantro and lime wedges. Add see salt and pepper to your liking.

Paleo Smoky Pork Tenderloin with Roasted Sweet Potatoes

Ingredients:

- 1 pound pork tenderloin
- 2 tsp. smoked paprika
- ¾ tsp. sea salt
- ½ tsp. ground black pepper
- ½ tsp. ground cumin
- 3 tbsp. virgin olive oil
- 2 large sweet potatoes peeled and cut
- ¼ cup apple cider vinegar
- 3 tbsp. maple syrup
- 1 tsp. mustard

Instructions:

Step 1: Preheat oven to 450 degrees F.

Step 2: Season the tenderloin with paprika, ¼ teaspoon salt, pepper, and cumin.

Step 3: Heat a large pan over medium heat and drizzle olive oil to the pan.

Step 4: Add the seasoned tenderloin to the pan and cook for 8 minutes, roughly 4 minutes on each side or until it comes to a nice brown char. The tenderloin doesn't need to be 100% cooked because we will bake it for 15 additional minutes.

Step 5: Put the potatoes and tenderloin on a baking sheet and drizzle with 1 tablespoon of olive oil. Bake them for 10-15 minutes.

Step 6: Remove the pan from the oven. Sprinkle the potatoes with ½ teaspoon of sea salt. Let it sit out for 5 minutes before cutting up into small pieces.

Step 7: Add the remaining 1/8 teaspoon salt, vinegar, maple syrup, mustard, and thyme in a small saucepan and bring it to a simmer.

Step 8: Drizzle over the potatoes and serve them with the tenderloin.

Eat up!

Chicken and Chile Hash

Ingredients:

- 2 tbsp. of water
- 12 ounces potatoes
- 2 tbsp. olive oil
- 1 tsp. sea salt
- ¼ tsp. ground red pepper
- 12 ounces of chicken
- 1 cup sliced red onion
- 1 poblano chile
- 2 cups cremini mushrooms
- 1 tbsp. chopped thyme
- 5 garlic cloves
- 3 tbsp. red wine vinegar
- 4 large eggs

Instructions:

Step 1: Put 2 tablespoons of water and potatoes in a microwave dish and cover them up with some plastic wrap. Microwave them for 5-7 minutes or until they get tender. After they are done, put them on a separate plate.

Step 2: Heat a large cooking pan over high heat and drizzle 1 tablespoon of olive oil.

Step 3: Season the chicken with ½ teaspoon salt, red pepper, and cook for 5 minutes and stir it to a crumble.

Step 4: Put the chicken mixture in a medium sized bowl.

Step 5: Add the onion and poblano chile to the pan and cook for 5 minutes. Add the mushrooms, 2 teaspoons thyme, and garlic and cook for another 5 minutes. Add mushroom mixture to the chicken.

Step 6: Add the remaining tablespoon of olive oil to the pan. Add the potatoes and cook for 5 minutes. Add the remaining ½ teaspoon salt, chicken mixture, and 1 tablespoon vinegar to the pan and cook for 5 more minutes.

Step 7: Fill a saucepan with water and bring it to a nice boil. Add the remaining 2 tablespoons of vinegar and reduce the heat. Break each egg into a cup, and pour each egg into the pan and cook for 3 minutes. After they are done cooking remove them from the pan.

Step 8: Serve each plate as you see fit and top with eggs and remaining teaspoon of thyme.

Enjoy!

Kale and Beet Salad with Salmon

Ingredients:

- 2/3 cup cider vinegar
- ½ cup water
- 1 tbsp. honey
- 1 cup red onion
- 4 beets
- 2 tbsp. olive oil
- 1 tsp. mustard
- ¼ tsp. sea salt
- ¼ tsp. black pepper
- 6 cups curly kale (torn)
- 2 boneless salmon (6-ounces each)
- ¼ cup sliced almonds

Instructions:

Step 1: Boil 2/3 cup vinegar, ½ cup water, and 2 teaspoons honey in a medium sized saucepan.

Step 2: Add the onion and boil for another 2-3 minutes. Turn the heat down and then lit it sit for 5 minutes.

Step 3: Microwave the beets on high for 5-7 minutes or until they get tender. After that, clean the beets and cut them into small wedge pieces.

Step 4: Mix the remaining 2 tablespoons of vinegar, remaining teaspoon of honey, oil, mustard, salt, and pepper in a large bowl.

Step 5: Add the beets and kale and cover them in the ingredients.

Step 6: Place 1 ½ cups kale mixture on each plate and top with 3 ounces of salmon, about ¼ cup onion, and 1 tablespoon of almonds or as you see fit.

Mushroom-Herb Chicken

Ingredients:

- 4 boneless chicken breasts (6-ounces each)
- ¼ tsp. sea salt
- ¼ tsp. black pepper
- 1 tsp. olive oil
- 3 large shallots
- 1 sliced mushroom (8-ounce)
- 1/3 cup red wine vinegar
- 1 tsp. dried marjoram
- 1 tsp. crushed ground black pepper

Instructions:

Step 1: Place each chicken breast half on 2 sheets of plastic wrap and pound them down with a meat mallet until they are about 1/3 inches thick.

Step 2: Season the chicken evenly with salt, ¼ teaspoon pepper and drizzle with ½ teaspoon olive oil.

Step 3: Heat up a large nonstick cooking pan over medium-high heat. Add the chicken to the cooking pan and cook it for 5 to 6 minutes on each side or until it turns golden brown.

Step 4: As the chicken cooks, cut up the three shallots into thin slices. When the chicken is done cooking remove it from the cooking pan and place on a separate plate.

Step 5: Cook the pan with ½ teaspoon of olive oil. Add the mushrooms and shallots to the pan and cook them for 2-3 minutes and stir them thoroughly. Add in the marjoram and continue stirring.

Step 6: Put the chicken back in the cooking pan and cover the pan. Cook it for another 5-7 minutes on medium heat with the mushrooms and shallots.

Step 7: After the chicken is done cooking, move it to a serving dish and enjoy. Add in ground pepper and salt if desired.

Grilled Scallop Salad

Ingredients:

- ½ tsp. ground black pepper
- ½ tsp. sea salt
- 12 sea scallops
- 1 sliced cucumber
- 2 tbsp. fresh lime juice
- 2 tsp. olive oil
- 4 cups romaine lettuce
- 3 cups watermelon
- ¼ cup fresh mint leaves
- ½ avocado

Instructions:

Step 1: Preheat the grill to medium-high heat and drizzle with some olive oil.

Step 2: Sprinkle ¼ teaspoon of pepper and ¼ teaspoon of salt over the scallops and cucumber. Arrange in a single layer on a grill rack coated with olive oil or cooking spray.

Step 3: Grill them for approximately 3 minutes on each side or until scallops are done and cucumber is well marked. Remove the scallops from the grill and cut the cucumber into small slices.

Step 4: Combine the remaining 1/8 teaspoon salt, juice, and oil in a large mixing bowl and stir it up. Add the cucumber, lettuce, watermelon, and the mint leaves and toss gently to coat.

Step 5: Divide the watermelon mixture evenly and top each serving with scallops and avocado slices. Sprinkle evenly with the remaining ¼ teaspoon freshly ground black pepper or as much as you prefer.

Eggs in Purgatory

Ingredients:

- 1 tbsp. olive oil
- 1 cup chopped onion
- 2 tsp. ground cumin
- 1 tsp. ground coriander
- 1 tsp. smoked paprika
- 1/8 tsp. ground cinnamon
- 4 garlic cloves
- 1 can crushed tomatoes
- 2 tbsp. harissa
- ¾ tsp. sea salt
- 8 large eggs (cage free)
- 1 package baby spinach (5-oz.)
- ¼ cup chopped cilantro

Instructions:

Step 1: Heat a large skillet over medium heat and drizzle oil to the pan.

Step 2: Add the onion, cumin, coriander, paprika, garlic, cinnamon and garlic and stir them until everything softens up and the flavor beings to pop.

Step 3: Stir in the crushed tomatoes, harissa, and ½ teaspoon salt. Cover and cook on high for roughly 20 minutes.

Step 4: After 20 minutes reduce the heat to low, and cook until the sauce is ready.

Step 5: One at a time, crack the eggs into a cooking pan and as they being to cook, slowly add in the prepped sauce. Cook on medium until everything has blended well.

Step 6: Season the eggs with the remaining ¼ teaspoon of sea salt and sprinkle cilantro on top.

Sweet Potato and Kale Masala Casserole

Ingredients:

For the Sauce:

- 2 tbsp. coconut oil
- 1 diced onion
- 1 serrano pepper
- 2 garlic cloves
- 1 tsp. ground ginger
- 1 tsp. ground cinnamon
- 1 tsp. ground cumin
- ½ tsp. coriander
- ½ tsp. turmeric
- ½ tsp. sea salt
- ½ tsp. black pepper
- 2 cups tomato puree
- 1 can of coconut milk
- ½ cup cilantro
- 1 medium lime

For the Casserole:

- 2 sweet potatoes
- 1 bunch stemmed kale (torn into small pieces)
- ¼ cup pepitas
- ¼ cup coconut flakes
- 2 tbsp. fresh cilantro
- 1/8 tsp. sea salt
- 1/8 tsp. black pepper

Instructions:

Step 1: Preheat oven to 375 degrees F.

Step 2: Make the sauce. Heat up the coconut oil in a deep cooking pan. Add in the onion and peppers and cook them until they get soft.

Step 3: Add in the garlic, ginger, and all of the seasonings and cook for about 3-5 minutes and stir actively. Put in the tomato puree and coconut milk, and simmer them for about 10 minutes. After that put in the lime juice and sprinkle in the cilantro.

Step 4: For the casserole, brush a casserole dish or ovenproof pan with some coconut oil.

Step 5: Put on the sliced sweet potatoes and kale and season with salt and pepper. Pour the masala sauce over the vegetables and cover the dish with tin-foil.

Step 6: Put this in the oven and bake for 40 minutes.

Step 7: After it is done baking, remove it from the oven and let it cool for 10 minutes before uncovering.

Step 8: Top with coconut flakes, cilantro and pepitas.

Eat up !

CHAPTER 8

PALEO SIDE DISHES AND SAUCES

Mini Parsnip Cakes with Buffalo Dip

Ingredients:

- 6 medium parsnips (1.5 pounds for 4 servings)
- 1 tsp. sea salt
- 1 large egg (cage free)
- ½ tsp. garlic powder
- ½ tsp. onion powder
- 1 tsp. coconut flour
- ½ tsp. black pepper
- ¼ cup olive oil
- ¼ cup mayonnaise
- 2 tsp. hot pepper sauce

Instructions:

Step 1: Place the parsnips in a medium-sized saucepan and cover them with cold water. Bring the water to a nice boil, and cook for 5-10 minutes. After they cook, drain them and allow them to cool.

Step 2: Once they have cooled, shred the parsnips on a box grater and lay on a separate plate. Season them with sea salt and let sit for 5 minutes.

Step 3: Squeeze out as much water as you can out of the parsnips and put them in a bowl.

Step 4: Add the egg, seasonings, and coconut flour and mix them well.

Step 5: Put the olive oil in a pan and heat to medium heat. When the oil beings to shimmer, place the parsnip mixture into the pan. Flatten slightly with a spatula and cook them until they are golden brown on both sides.

Step 6: Mix up the mayo with the hot sauce and serve as a side.

Sweet Potato Casserole

Ingredients:

For the Sweet Potatoes:

- 6 peeled sweet potatoes
- ½ cup coconut milk
- 2 tbsp. coconut oil
- 1 orange (squeezed)
- 1 tsp. ginger
- 1 tsp. cinnamon
- 1 tsp. sea salt

For the Toppings:

- 1 cup of pecans
- 1 tsp. cinnamon
- 2 tbsp. maple syrup
- 1 tbsp. of melted coconut oil
- ½ tsp. sea salt

Instructions:

Step 1: Preheat oven to 350 degrees F.

Step 2: Put the potatoes in a saucepan and cover them with cold water. Bring to a boil, reduce to a simmer, and cook for 10-12 minutes or until tender. Drain the potatoes after.

Step 3: Move the potatoes to a large bowl and mash well with a potato masher.

Step 4: Add the coconut milk, coconut oil, orange juice and zest, ginger, cinnamon, and salt. Mix well, and spread into a casserole dish.

Step 5: Combine the ingredient for the topping in a bowl until the pecans are well coated. Spread them over the potatoes and bake them for 15 minutes.

Step 6: If desired, turn the broiler on to a high heat and broil until the topping is well browned before serving.

Apple Beet and Arugula Salad

Ingredients:

- 3 large beets
- 3 granny smith apples (peeled)
- ¾ cup raw pecans (chopped)
- 3 ½ packed cups of baby arugula, lightly chopped
- ½ orange (juiced)
- 2 tbsp. olive oil
- 1 tbsp. apple cider vinegar
- 1-2 tbsp. raw honey
- Sea salt
- Ground black pepper

Instructions:

Step 1: Preheat oven to 400 degrees F.

Step 2: Wash and dry beets and leave the skin on. Drizzle some olive oil over each beet and sprinkle each with a pinch of sea salt.

Step 3: Wrap each beet in aluminum foil and put them on a baking sheet. Bake them for roughly 60 minutes or until they are ready.

Step 4: Take the beets out of the oven and allow them to cool down for about 5-10 minutes. Unwrap each beet and drain the excess beet juice into a small bowl and set aside.

Step 5: Slice the beets into small pieces and place in a large mixing bowl.

Step 6: Fill the bottom of a medium sized cooking pan with water and place a steamer basket in it.

Step 7: Place over medium-high heat and bring the water to a nice boil. Add the chopped apples, cover and steam them for about 4-5 minutes or until the apples are soft and tender. Drain and add the steamed apples to the bowl with the beets.

144

Step 8: Place ¾ cup of chopped pecans in a medium sized skillet over medium-heat and cook until lightly toasted, stirring frequently. Set the pecans aside.

Step 9: To make the dressing, take the left-over beet juice and add the 2 tablespoons of olive, apple cider vinegar, raw honey, orange juice and orange zest.

Step 10: Stir it and add sea salt and black pepper to your liking. Pour the dressing over the beet mixture and toss to coat. Add the arugula and toasted pecans and toss again.

Paleo Baked Butternut Squash

Ingredients:

- 3 pounds butternut squash (peeled and cut into small pieces)
- 3 tbsp. olive oil
- 1 ½ tbsp. balsamic vinegar
- 2 tsp. sea salt
- 1 tsp. ground black pepper

Instructions:

Step 1: Preheat oven to 400 degrees F.

Step 2: Place the butternut squash in a bowl and toss to coat with olive oil, vinegar, salt and pepper.

Step 3: Dump the squash onto the baking sheet and arrange into a single layer.

Step 4: Bake for 30 minutes, stirring with a spatula a couple times during baking.

Step 5: Taste and add additional sea salt or ground black pepper if needed.

Paleo Cauliflower Fried Rice

Ingredients:

- 1 head of cauliflower
- 3 tbsp. bacon fat
- 4 medium sized carrots
- 1 chopped onion
- 2 cloves of garlic
- 1 cup green peas
- 4 large eggs (cage free)
- 6 tbsp. coconut aminos
- ½ tsp. sesame oil
- ½ tsp. fish sauce

Instructions:

Step 1: Chop up the cauliflower into small florets. Put some florets into the food processor or blender and pulse 2 or 3 times or until the rice sized pieces begin to form.

Step 2: Put them in a large mixing bowl and continue until all of the cauliflower turns to a rice like texture. Wrap up the riced cauliflower in some paper towels and drain out any additional moisture and after that put back in the mixing bowl.

Step 3: Heat up a cooking pan on medium-high heat and add 2 tablespoons of bacon fat and let it melt.

Step 4: Add the onions, carrots and garlic and cook for about 3-5 minutes. Add the green peas, cook for another extra 2-3 minutes. Remove them from the pan and set aside in a medium sized bowl.

Step 5: Add the four eggs to the pan and scramble them until they are lightly browned. Add a pinch of sea salt and pepper, then move the food from the pan into the bowl with the veggies and set aside.

Step 6: Add the remaining tablespoons of bacon fat to the pan and coat it evenly. Heat up the pan until it gets hot.

Step 7: Add cauliflower to the pan and toss it lightly. Cook it for about 5-7 minutes or until the pieces become light brown and slightly crispy.

Step 8: Add the veggie and rice mixture back to the pan and stir to combine. Add the sesame oil, coconut aminos, fish sauce and stir to combine. After the flavors blend and get done cooking, serve immediately.

Enjoy!

Paleo Coleslaw

Ingredients:

- 2 bags of pre-made coleslaw or large sliced cabbage

For the dressing:

- ½ cup raw honey
- ½ cup apple cider vinegar
- 1/3 cup light tasting olive oil
- ½ tsp. sea salt
- ½ tsp. dry mustard
- ½ tsp. celery seed
- ½ tsp. garlic powder
- ½ tsp. ground black pepper

Instructions:

Step 1: Heat up a medium-sized cooking pan and add all the dressing ingredients to the pan. Bring it to a nice simmer and stir for about 5-6 minutes.

Step 2: Pour the dressing over the coleslaw mix and toss to coat. Cover and place in the refrigerator for at least one hour or until chilled. Taste and adjust any seasonings as needed.

Paleo Crispy Brussel Sprouts

Ingredients:

- ¾ pounds of brussels sprouts
- 1 ½ tbsp. olive oil
- ¼ tsp. sea salt
- ¼ tsp. ground black pepper

Instructions:

Step 1: Preheat oven to 400 degrees F.

Step 2: Cut the brussels sprouts in half and place them in a medium sized bowl. Drizzle the olive oil over the brussels sprouts and toss in a pinch of sea salt and black pepper until they are evenly coated.

Step 3: Get a baking sheet and place the brussels sprouts on it.

Step 4: Bake them for 10-15 minutes and serve as a side dish or enjoy as a nice little snack. Add conservative amounts of sea salt and pepper if you desire

Paleo Muffins

Ingredients:

- ½ cup coconut flour
- 2 tsp. baking powder
- ½ tsp. sea salt
- 4 eggs (cage free)
- 2 tsp. apple cider vinegar
- 2 ½ tbsp. unsweetened applesauce
- 1 ½ tbsp. raw honey
- ½ cup coconut oil or ghee
- Raw honey

Instructions:

Step 1: Preheat oven to 350 degrees F.

Step 2: Mix in the coconut flour, baking powder and sea salt together in a medium sized mixing bowl. Set it to the side.

Step 3: Mix the eggs, vinegar and applesauce in a food processor or blender for roughly 15 seconds. Add in some honey and coconut oil and blend for another 15 seconds.

Step 4: Add the dry ingredients and blend them until they are well mixed.

Step 5: Pour the mixture in a muffin tin and fill each one about ¾ of the way full. You should be able to make roughly 10 muffins.

Step 6: Bake the muffins for 20-25 minutes. Take them out of the oven and allow them to sit for 5-10 minutes before removing from the muffin tin and serving.

Yummy !!!

Paleo Greens and Ham Hock

Ingredients:

- 1 large smoked ham hock
- 3 bunches of collard greens
- 6 slices of bacon
- 1 tbsp. bacon fat
- 1 chopped sweet onion
- 6 cloves of garlic
- 1 tsp. sea salt
- ¾ tsp. pepper

Instructions:

Step 1: Put 7 cups of water and ham hock in a large saucepan and bring the water to a nice even boil.

Step 2: Turn down the heat to low and let it simmer for approximately 1 hour. Remove any scrum from the water and discard.

Step 3: Take the ham hock out but don't dump the water. Put the ham hock and saucepan to the side.

Step 4: Cut up the ham hock meat and remove the skin and bones.

Step 5: Cook the bacon in a large pot on medium heat until it gets nice and crispy. After it is done cooking remove the bacon and set it to the side. Drain the bacon fat from the pan and leave 3 tablespoons in the pan.

Step 6: Add in the onion and sauté for about 5 minutes. After that add in the garlic and ham hock and sauté for another 2-3 minutes.

Step 7: Measure 3 ½ cups of the ham hock broth and add it to the stockpot and bring it to a light boil until they mix well.

Step 8: Reduce the heat to low, add the salt and pepper, and allow the collard greens to cook for 1 hour while stirring consistently. Add in the bacon to the pot and cook for another 30 minutes.

Paleo Hasselback Sweet Potatoes

Ingredients:

- 1lb sweet potatoes
- 1 tsp. sea salt
- 2 tbsp. ghee (30g)
- 1 clove of chopped garlic
- 1 tsp. chopped rosemary
- 1 tsp. thyme

Instructions:

Step 1: Preheat the oven to 375 degrees F.

Step 2: Line a baking sheet with some tin-foil. Peel the skin off the sweet potatoes and then cut up the sweet potatoes into thin slices.

Step 3: Put the sweet potatoes on the baking sheet and drizzle them with the ghee and add a pinch of salt to the top. Bake them for 60 to 70 minutes or until the sweet potatoes are nice and soft.

Step 4: In a separate mixing bowl, mix in the remaining ghee and combine it with chopped rosemary, garlic and thyme. Stir it thoroughly until it forms a nice and soft mixture.

Step 5: Drizzle the sweet potatoes with the mix.

Paleo Italian Breaded Eggplant

Ingredients:

- 1 eggplant sliced into thin pieces
- 1 large egg (cage free)
- ¼ cup flour
- ½ tsp. sea salt
- ¼ tsp. ground black pepper
- ¼ tsp. oregano
- ¼ tsp. thyme
- ¼ tsp. garlic powder
- Bacon fat
- Marinara sauce
- Chopped parsley (optional)
- Cooling rack
- Paper towels and some plates

Instructions:

Step 1: Put the eggplant in a strainer and toss with some sea salt. Let it sit for 20-25 minutes to drain. This will remove the excess moisture.

Step 2: Put the egg in a bowl and whisk it thoroughly. Put the arrowroot flour in a separate bowl and add the sea salt, black pepper, oregano, thyme and garlic powder, and stir them thoroughly.

Step 3: Rinse off the eggplant and dry it with some paper towels.

Step 4: Dip the eggplant slices in the egg mix and then into the arrowroot flour mixture and make sure to coat each side evenly.

Step 5: Place the eggplant slices on a cooling rack and continue to dip the rest until they are all evenly coated.

Step 6: Cover a medium sized cooking pan with bacon fat and heat the pan up.

Step 7: Fry the eggplant slices for roughly 2-3 minutes on each side or until the sides begin to get golden crispy.

Step 8: After they are done frying, move the eggplants to a plate lined with paper towels and allow them to cool off and for some of the fat to get absorbed.

Step 9: Serve them on a separate plate with marinara sauce on the side for dipping.

Enjoy!

Paleo Breadsticks

Ingredients:

- 1 ½ cup almond flour
- ½ cup tapioca flour
- 1 tsp. baking powder
- ½ tsp. salt
- 2 eggs (cage free)
- 2 tbsp. virgin olive oil
- 1 ½ tbsp. ghee
- ½ tsp. garlic powder
- ¼ tsp. freshly chopped parsley
- Marinara sauce (for dipping)

Instructions:

Step 1: Preheat oven to 400 degrees F.

Step 2: Take the almond flour, tapioca flour, baking powder and sea salt and place them in a medium-sized mixing bowl and stir them until they are well mixed. After you have mixed the ingredients, put them to the side.

Step 3: In a separate mixing bowl, add the eggs and whisk them well. After that add in the olive oil and whisk them until they are well combined.

Step 4: After that, pour the egg mixture into the flour mixture and mix it until dough begins to form. You may need to add additional water or flour until you get a nice smooth dough. Knead the dough until it is no longer sticky.

Step 5: Split up the dough into 10-12 sized balls, and then roll them in a 9" rope. Take two separate pieces of rope and lace them around each other to form the twist shape. Set those on a baking sheet and continue with the rest of the ropes.

Step 6: Place the pan into the oven and bake them for 8-10 minutes.

Step 7: While the breadsticks are baking, warm up the ghee, garlic powder and ¼ tsp. sea salt and stir them until they combine well.

Step 8: After the breadsticks are done cooking, remove them from the oven and drizzle them with the ghee mixture. After that put them back in the oven for an additional 2-3 minutes.

Step 9: After that take them out of the oven and sprinkle some dried parsley and let it sit for 2-3 minutes. Serve the breadsticks with some marinara sauce for dipping.

Paleo Orange and Ginger Glazed Carrots

Ingredients:

- 1lb. peeled carrots
- 1 cup water
- Pinch of sea salt
- 1 tbsp. ghee
- 1 juiced orange
- 2 tbsp. honey
- ½ tsp. ground ginger
- Ground black pepper
- Lemon zest

Instructions:

Step 1: Place water some sea salt in a medium-sized saucepan and add the carrots. Bring the water to an even boil and reduce the heat to medium and wait until the carrots being to soften up. Once the carrots are soft, dump out the excess water.

Step 2: Add the ghee, orange juice, lemon zest, honey, ginger and pepper to the pan. Stir to combine the flavors with the carrots and sauté for another 5 minutes until the carrots are tender and the glaze has thickened slightly.

Paleo Bacon Wrapped Asparagus

Ingredients:

- 1 lb. of asparagus
- 10 pieces of bacon
- 1 tbsp. balsamic vinegar
- 1 tbsp. extra virgin olive oil
- Black pepper
- 1 lemon

Instructions:

Step 1: Preheat oven to 400 degrees F.

Step 2: Wrap one half-slice of bacon tightly around each piece of asparagus and place on a baking sheet covered in aluminum foil.

Step 3: Drizzle balsamic vinegar and olive oil over the asparagus and sprinkle with a pinch of ground black pepper.

Step 4: Bake for 15 minutes, then flip each asparagus over and bake for another 10-15 minutes or until the bacon is nice and crispy.

Step 5: Serve right away with lemon wedges on the side.

Paleo Red Cabbage

Ingredients:

- 3 tbsp. ghee
- ¼ cup chopped sweet onion
- 1 large head of red cabbage
- 2 peeled green apples (sliced into thin pieces)
- ¼ cup water
- 1/3 cup apple cider vinegar
- ¼ cup raw honey

Instructions:

Step 1: Place a large cooking pan over medium heat and add the ghee until it melts. After it melts add the chopped onion and cook for another 3-5 minutes. Add the rest of the ingredients and stir to combine them.

Step 2: Add the cabbage and sliced green apples and bring everything to a nice boil then reduce the heat to low.

Step 3: Cover it and let it simmer for 1 ½ hours or until the cabbage is soft and tender.

Taste and add additional salt or black pepper if needed.

Paleo Sautéed Balsamic Mushrooms

Ingredients:

- 1lb. white button mushrooms
- 3 tbsp. bacon fat
- 1 chopped white onion
- 2 chopped garlic cloves
- ½ tsp. sea salt
- ¼ tsp. ground black pepper
- 1 ½ tbsp. balsamic vinegar
- 1 tbsp. chopped parsley (optional)

Instructions:

Step 1: Clean off the mushrooms and then slice them in half and set them aside.

Step 2: Put the bacon fat in a large pan and place on medium heat. Let the fat melt, then add the mushrooms, onion and garlic and simmer for about 8-10 minutes or until the mushrooms are nice and tender.

Step 3: Add the sea salt, pepper and balsamic vinegar to the pan and stir it evenly. Cook for another 2-5 minutes.

Serve with a dash of chopped parsley if desired.

Paleo Sesame Noodles

Ingredients:

- 1 package kelp noodles
- ½ tbsp. bacon fat
- 2 cloves of chopped garlic
- Hint of red pepper flakes
- 1/3 cup almond butter
- 1 can coconut milk (14 oz)
- 1 tbsp. sesame oil
- 1 tbsp. raw honey
- 2 tbsp. coconut aminos
- Sea salt and ground black pepper

Instructions:

Step 1: Place a large saucepan half-filled with water over medium-heat and bring to a boil.

Step 2: Add the noodles and let them cook until they become nice and tender. Usually takes 20-25 minutes.

Step 3: In a separate pan, add the bacon fat and set to medium-heat and then add the garlic and sauté for 2-3 minutes. After that add the red pepper flakes and stir evenly until the flavors combine.

Step 4: Add almond butter, coconut milk, sesame oil, raw honey and coconut aminos and stir them until they are evenly combined. Bring them to a boil and then reduce the heat to low.

Step 5: Allow time for the sauce to reduce and stir it frequently for about 20 minutes or so.

Step 6: Once the noodles are done cooking, drain them and put them back in the pan. Add the sauce and toss the noodles until they are fully coated.

Paleo Spicy Smashed Sweet Potatoes

Ingredients:

- 3 sweet potatoes
- ½ tsp. chili powder
- ½ tsp. cumin
- ½ tsp. garlic powder
- ½ tsp. onion powder
- ½ tsp. paprika
- ½ tsp. sea salt
- 1/8 tsp. ground black pepper

For the Sauce:

- 1 tbsp. raw honey
- 2 tbsp. olive oil

Instructions:

Step 1: Preheat oven to 400 degrees F.

Step 2: In a medium sized bowl mix together all ingredients for the spice mixture and set aside.

Step 3: Poke some holes in each sweet potato and place directly on the oven rack. Cook them for 25-35 minutes or until the sweet potatoes are nice and tender.

Step 4: Once the potatoes are done take them out of the oven, turn the oven to broil, and then peel off the skin.

Step 5: Cut the potatoes into thin slices and place them on a cookie sheet.

Step 6: Take a cup and gently press down on each sweet potato circle until the side's split open. This will allow the edges to get nice and crispy later.

Step 7: Mix the raw honey and olive oil in a separate bowl and use half of the mixture to drizzle over all of the sweet potatoes. Take half of your spice mixture and sprinkle some over each sweet potato.

Step 8: Put the potatoes back into the oven and broil for 5 minutes. Be careful not to burn them.

Step 9: Take the pan out and flip each potato over. Drizzle the remaining sauce over the sweet potatoes and add the remaining spices.

Enjoy!

CHAPTER 9

PALEO DESSERTS AND SNACKS

Chocolate Hazelnut Tart

Ingredients:

- Foil-lined muffin cups or tins

For the Crust:

- ¾ cups hazelnut flour
- 2 tsp. cocoa powder
- 3 tbsp. coconut oil
- 1 tbsp. maple syrup
- 1/8 tsp. sea salt

For the Filling:

- 3 tbsp. coconut oil
- 3 tbsp. coconut milk
- 3 tbsp. maple syrup
- 6 tbsp. cocoa powder
- ½ tsp. vanilla extract

Instructions:

For the Tart Molds:

Step 1: Use foil or muffing cups and place a regular-mouth mason jar top-down in the center of the muffin liner and press down until the liner becomes wider.

For the crust:

Step 1: Combine all the crust ingredients in a medium sized bowl and stir evenly until they are well combined.

Step 2: Split the mixture into quarters and press evenly into the bottom sides of the prepared tart molds.

Step 3: Set the crusts in a baking pan with a flat bottom and set aside while you prepare the filling.

For the Filling:

Step 1: Heat up coconut milk, coconut oil, and maple syrup in a medium sized saucepan until it becomes nice and smooth. Don't let it simmer or come to a boil.

Step 2: Turn the heat to low and stir in the cocoa powder and vanilla extract until smooth.

Step 3: Pour the filling mixture evenly between the prepared tart molds.

Step 4: Put the tart molds in the refrigerator to chill them for at least 1 hour or until they become firm.

Step 5: Serve them with strawberries, cocoa powder, and hazelnuts on top if desired.

Chocolate Chip Paleo Zucchini Bread

Ingredients:

- 1 cup shredded zucchini
- 1 ripe banana
- 6 eggs (cage free)
- 3 tbsp. maple syrup
- 2 tbsp. coconut oil
- 1 tsp. vanilla extract
- ¾ cup coconut flour
- 1 ½ tsp. ground cinnamon
- ¾ tsp. baking soda
- ¼ tsp. ground nutmeg
- 1/8 tsp. sea salt
- 4 ounces dark chocolate

Instructions:

Step 1: Preheat oven to 350 degrees F.

Step 2: Prep a metal baking pan with parchment paper and allow it to hang over the two sides.

Step 3: Put the shredded zucchini between two paper towels and press out as much water as you can.

Step 4: In a large bowl, mash the banana, whisk in the eggs, maple syrup, coconut oil, and vanilla. Sprinkle in the coconut flour, cinnamon, baking soda, nutmeg, and salt, then stir it until evenly combined.

Step 5: Stir in the shredded zucchini, then fold in two-thirds of the chocolate. Pour the batter into the prepared pan and gently smooth the top. Sprinkle the remaining third of the chocolate on top.

Step 6: Bake for 30 to 35 minutes or until the top is golden.

Step 7: Take it out of the oven and let it cool on a rack for 25-30 minutes. After it cools, slowly remove the bread from the pan.

Enjoy!

Pumpkin Donut Holes

Ingredients:

For the donut holes:

- ½ cup coconut flour (60 grams)
- ¾ cup almond flour (70 grams)
- 1 ¼ tsp. baking soda
- 3 ½ tsp. pumpkin pie spice
- ¼ tsp. sea salt
- 4 large eggs (cage free)
- 6 tbsp. of unsalted butter or coconut oil (98 grams)
- ½ cup of maple syrup
- 2 tbsp. brown sugar
- ½ cup canned pumpkin puree
- 2 tsp. vanilla extract

For the cinnamon sugar:

- 1/3 cup coconut sugar (60 grams)
- 1 ½ tsp. ground cinnamon

Instructions:

Step 1: Preheat oven to 400 degrees F.

Step 2: Line a muffin pan with muffin liners.

Step 3: In a large bowl, mix together all the dry ingredients.

Step 4: In a separate medium-sized bowl, mix together the wet ingredients. After that add the dry mixture to the wet mixture and stir it until it's well combined.

Step 5: Pour the batter evenly into the muffin liners, filling each liner until almost completely full.

Step 6: Bake for 10-15 minutes. Turn out onto a wire rack to cool completely. These need to rest for at least an hour before serving.

Step 7: When ready to serve, mix the cinnamon with the sugar in a small bowl.

Step 8: Roll the donut holes in the cinnamon sugar. As these donut holes are quite moist, the cinnamon sugar tends to liquify overnight, which is why it's recommended to roll the donuts in the sugar no more than 8 hours before serving.

Store in a container for up to 2 days.

Chocolate Chip Coconut Flour Pumpkin Bars

Ingredients:

- 1 cup canned pumpkin puree
- ¼ cup puree maple syrup
- 1 tsp. vanilla extract
- ¼ cup almond butter
- 1 tsp. unsweetened almond milk
- 2 eggs (cage free)
- ½ cup coconut flour
- ¾ tsp. baking soda
- 1/8 tsp. sea salt
- 1 tsp. cinnamon
- ½ tsp. ginger
- ¼ tsp. nutmeg
- 1/8 tsp. ground cloves
- ½ cup chocolate chips

Instructions:

Step 1: Preheat oven to 400 degrees F.

Step 2: Line a baking pan with parchment paper and spray it down with cooking spray.

Step 3: Add pumpkin puree, maple syrup, vanilla extract, almond butter, almond milk and eggs to a large bowl and mix until well combined, smooth and creamy.

Step 4: Add coconut flour, baking soda, salt and the rest of remaining spices. Gently fold in 1/3 cup of chocolate chips into the batter. Spread batter evenly in prepared pan.

Step 5: Bake for 20-25 minutes. Move the pan to a wire rack to cool.

Step 6: Melt the remaining ¼ cup of chocolate chip in a small saucepan over low heat. Once the chocolate is completely melted, drizzle it over the bars.

Paleo Carrot Cake Loaf

Ingredients:

- 2 cups almond flour
- 3 tsp. coconut flour
- 3 eggs (cage free)
- 2 tbsp. coconut oil
- 1/3 cup apple sauce
- 1/3 cup grated carrots
- 1 tsp. organic vanilla extract
- 1/8 tsp. Himalayan sea salt
- ½ tsp. cinnamon
- 1 tsp. baking soda
- 1 tsp. baking powder

Optional: mini chocolate chips, raisins, walnuts

Instructions:

Step 1: Preheat oven to 350 degrees F.

Step 2: Mix the dry ingredients in a medium sized mixing bowl.

Step 3: Add in wet ingredients and mix well with the dry ingredients.

Step 4: Add in carrots and optional ingredients.

Step 5: Grease a bread pan and pour in the batter.

Step 6: Bake for 20-25 minutes.

Vanilla Cake

Ingredients:

For the cake:

- 4 eggs (cage free)
- 4 tbsp. raw honey
- 5 tbsp. coconut flour
- 5 tbsp. almond flour
- ½ tsp. baking powder
- 1/8 tsp. sea salt

For the filing:

- 1 ¾ cups raw cashews
- ¼ cup coconut oil
- 1/3 cup honey
- 1/3 cup of water
- ½ tsp. lemon juice
- 1/8 tsp. sea salt
- 1 tbsp. sliced almonds (optional)

Instructions:

*** Make the filling a day ahead ***

Step 1: Put all the ingredients besides the water in a blender and blend them until they become smooth. After that add the water, a tablespoon at a time until the filling becomes nice and smooth.

Step 2: Move the filling to a bowl, cover with plastic wrap and chill overnight.

Step 3: To make the cake, preheat the oven to 350 degrees F.

Step 4: Line two spring-form pans with parchment paper.

Step 5: In a large bowl mix the eggs with honey. Add the salt, coconut flour mixed with baking powder and seeds from vanilla pod and mix until well combined.

Step 6: Split the mixture between the prepared pans and bake for 15-20 minutes. After they are done baking, remove the cakes from the oven and set aside to cool.

Step 7: Remove the cakes from the pans and get the filling from the fridge. Whip the filling with a hand mixer until filling becomes fluffy.

Step 8: Put one of the cakes on a platter and spread 1/3 of the filling evenly. Top with another cake and spread top and sides of cake with remaining filling.

Paleo Edible Chocolate Chip Cookie Dough

Ingredients:

- ½ cup packed almond flour
- ¼ cup tapioca flour
- 5 tbsp. butter
- 2-3 tsp. of honey
- ¾ tsp. vanilla
- 1-ounce dark chocolate
- Pinch of sea salt

Instructions:

Step 1: Combine all ingredients in a blender and blend until they get smooth.

Step 2: Taste and see if you need more honey, vanilla, or salt depending on your taste. If you do, just add a little bit at a time until its ready.

Add in the chocolate and serve.

Death Cookies (don't let the name scare you)

Ingredients:

- 1 cup mashed banana
- 2 eggs (cage free)
- 2 tsp. vanilla extract
- 2 tbsp. coconut milk or coconut water
- ½ cup chocolate chips
- 1 cup cocoa powder
- ¼ cup honey
- ½ tsp. baking soda

Instructions:

Step 1: Preheat oven to 350 degrees F.

Step 2: Place everything in a blender except baking soda and puree until smooth.

Step 3: Put in the baking soda and spread batter into prepared dish.

Step 4: Bake for 25-30 minutes.

Step 5: Let the cookies cool for about 10 minutes before removing. Add in the chocolate chips and serve.

Coconut Crack Bars

Ingredients:

- 1 cup shredded coconut (85g)
- ¼ cup agave or pure maple syrup
- 2 tbsp. coconut
- ½ tsp pure vanilla extract
- Raw chocolate chips (optional)

Instructions:

Step 1: Mix all the ingredients in a food processor or blender.

Step 2: Put into a small container and put in the fridge for an hour before trying to cut.

Step 3: Once they have cooled, take them out of the fridge and cut them up.

Banana Pudding

Ingredients:

- 4 egg yolks
- ¼ cup honey
- ¼ cup arrowroot powder
- 2 ripe bananas
- ½ tsp. sea salt
- 2 cups full-fat coconut milk
- 1 tsp. vanilla extract
- Walnuts

Instructions:

Step 1: Mix together the egg yolks, honey, and arrowroot powder in a medium sized bowl and then set aside.

Step 2: Heat up the coconut milk in a medium sized saucepan and stir occasionally for 5 minutes. Slowly pour the coconut milk into the egg mix and whisk consistently.

Step 3: Put the entire mixture back into the saucepan and cook for another 3-5 minutes. Stir regularly until it gets thick and make sure it does not come to a boil.

Step 4: Move the mixture into a large bowl and mix in the vanilla and the mashed bananas. Let it chill for one hour.

Step 5: To serve, spoon the pudding into a glass. Top it with a sliced banana and walnuts if desired.

Lemon Berry Skillet Cake

Ingredients:

- 1/2 cup coconut flour
- ¼ tsp. sea salt
- ½ tsp. baking soda
- 6 eggs (cage free)
- 6 tbsp. maple syrup
- ½ cup coconut oil
- 6 tbsp. coconut
- 1 tsp. vanilla extract
- 1 tbsp. lemon juice
- 1 cup of mixed berries
- Coconut oil

Instructions:

Step 1: Preheat the oven to 350 degrees F.

Step 2: Mix together the coconut flour, sea salt, baking soda and set it aside.

Step 3: Whisk the eggs until they are nice and foamy. After that add in the coconut oil, coconut milk, vanilla, and lemon juice. Mix thoroughly to combine.

Step 4: Add the dry ingredients to the wet ingredients and mix them until they are well combined. Let them sit for 2-3 minutes to allow the coconut flour to absorb.

Step 5: Pour the mix into the greased skillet. Gently spread evenly across the bottom of the skillet. Add the berries on top.

Step 6: Bake them for 25-30 minutes or until the cake comes to a light gold color.

Enjoy!

Pecan Snowball Cookies

Ingredients:

- 1 cup pecan halves
- ½ cup shredded coconut
- 1 cup soft dates
- 1 tbsp. coconut oil
- ½ tsp. sea salt
- ½ tsp. vanilla extract
- ½ cup arrowroot

Instructions:

Step 1: Preheat the oven to 375 degrees F.

Step 2: Line a baking sheet with parchment paper and set it aside.

Step 3: Put the pecans and shredded coconut in a blender or food processor and blend until the pecans are finely ground. Add all of the remaining ingredients and process until a sticky dough is formed.

Step 4: Scoop a few tablespoons full of dough and shape into small round balls, then place them on a prepared baking sheet.

Step 5: Bake them for 12-15 minutes or until you notice a light brown color.

Paleo Strawberry Crumble

Ingredients:

For the filling:

- 4 cups of strawberries
- 2 tbsp. tapioca flour
- 2 tsp. vanilla extract
- 1 tbsp. fresh lemon juice
- 2 tbsp. maple syrup

For the Crumble Topping:

- 1 cup almond flour
- ½ tsp. sea salt
- 3 tbsp. coconut oil
- 3 tbsp. pure maple syrup

Instructions:

Step 1: Preheat the oven to 350 degrees F.

Step 2: In a mixing bowl, toss together the strawberries, tapioca flour, vanilla extract, lemon juice, and maple syrup.

Step 3: Move everything to the baking pan

Step 4: Mix together the ingredients for the crumble topping in a medium sized bowl.

Step 5: Spread it evenly over the strawberries and bake in the oven for 30 minutes.

Step 6: After it is done cooking, let it stand for 10 minutes before serving with ice cream.

Non-Dairy & Paleo Strawberry Cheesecake

(This is an involved process, but its so worth it)

Ingredients:

For the Crust:

- 140g of shredded unsweetened coconut
- 90g raw hazelnuts
- 30g (1/4 cup) coconut flour
- ¼ cup coconut oil
- 2 tbsp. raw honey
- 1 tbsp. blackstrap molasses
- 1 tsp. sea salt
- ½ tsp. ground ginger
- ½ tsp. ground cinnamon

For the Filling:

- 300g (2 cups) raw cashew pieces
- 1 cup coconut milk
- 1 pound of cauliflower
- 1 cup of honey
- ¾ cup coconut oil
- 1 tsp. sea salt
- ½ tsp. ground cinnamon
- 1 tbsp. apple cider vinegar
- 1 tbsp. vanilla extract
- 6 eggs (cage free)
- Lemon zest
- ¼ cup tapioca flour

For the Garnish:

- 4 cups fresh strawberries
- 1 tbsp. grass-fed gelatin
- ½ cup cold water
- ½ cup water

- 2 tbsp. pure maple syrup
- Pinch of sea salt
- ½ tsp. pure vanilla extract

Instructions:

FOR THE CRUST:

Step 1: Line the bottom of a springform pan with parchment paper.

Step 2: Grease the side of the pan with coconut oil.

Step 3: Add in all the ingredients for the crust to your food processor or blender and process until the mixture has been fully mixed.

Step 4: Press at the bottom and side of the pan. You want to bring the crust up to about halfway up the side of the pan.

FOR THE FILLING:

Step 1: Preheat the oven to 350 degrees F.

Step 2: Use a large size cheese grater of your choice and grate the cauliflower.

Step 3: Place the grated cauliflower in a microwaveable bowl and cover it loosely with plastic film and microwave for about 5 minutes on high.

Step 4: Let the cauliflower cool for 5 minutes.

Step 5: After is has cooled, squeeze it as dry as you can.

Step 6: After that boil 3-4 cups of water.

Step 7: Rinse the cashew pieces under running cold water and add them to the mix along with the coconut milk to the bowl of your food processor or blender. Process the mix until everything is nice and creamy.

Step 8: Add honey, coconut oil, salt, cinnamon, apple cider vinegar and vanilla and then resume processing until well combined for roughly 1-2 minutes.

Step 9: Throw in the lemon zest and juice and mix until they are well combined. After that add the eggs one at a time and mix for about 30 seconds between each addition.

Step 10: Add tapioca flour and give your filling a final 30 second spin. After that pour it over the reserved crust.

Step 11: Place the cake over a piece of aluminum foil and fold it over around the pan.

Step 12: Place your cake in a pan then pour boiling water into the pan so it goes to about ¼ of the way full. Place that rig onto the middle rack of your oven and bake for 15 minutes then lower the temperature to 250 degrees F and bake for another 90 minutes.

Step 13: Turn off the oven and open it. Let the cake cool off in the oven for about 1 hour and then slide it out of the oven.

Step 14: When the cheesecake has cooled off, run a knife around the rim and refrigerate uncovered for at least 5-6 hours.

FOR THE GARNISH

Step 1: Sprinkle the gelatin over ½ cups of cold water and let it rest for a few minutes to allow the gelatin to soak up as much water as possible.

Step 2: At the same time boil 1 cup of strawberries and half a cup of water in a small cooking pan. Let that boil for about 5-7 minutes or until the strawberries have released their red color to the water.

Step 3: After that, strain them through a sieve right over the gelatin and stir until the gelatin is completely dissolved.

Step 4: Next, stir in the maple syrup, vanilla extract and salt and let this mixture cool until it starts to set. Placing it in the fridge will speed up the process.

Step 5: While your strawberry jelly is setting, arrange the strawberries over the top of your cake and cover it completely.

Step 6: Add the strawberry jelly over the strawberries with a pastry brush.

Step 7: Place the cake in the fridge until the jelly is completely set, roughly for about 1 hour and then serve.

Pecan Pie Ice Cream

Ingredients:

- 1.5 cups of raw pecans
- 1 tbsp. coconut sugar
- 2 tsp. coconut oil
- ¾ cup almond milk
- 3 ¼ cups coconut cream
- 1/3 cup pure maple syrup
- 2 tsp. vanilla extract
- 2 tsp. molasses (optional)
- 1 tbsp. bourbon (optional)

Instructions:

Step 1: Preheat the oven to 325 degrees F.

Step 2: Toss your pecans in 1 tablespoon of coconut sugar and coconut oil and then bake it until it becomes nicely roasted.

Step 3: Remove from the oven and set aside to cool.

Step 4: In a small cooking pan, warm the almond milk with the remaining coconut sugar and stir until fully dissolved. Don't overheat the milk, you just want it warm enough to dissolve the sugar.

Step 5: In a large mixing bowl, add in the almond milk, coconut cream, maple syrup, vanilla, molasses and bourbon. Whisk all the ingredients until they are well combined. Add more salt and more maple if needed.

Step 6: Next, chop up the pecans.

Step 7: Churn the ice cream per manufacturer's instructions. In the last stages of churning add the toasted pecans. Once churned, put into a freezer-safe container and freeze until nice and firm.

Step 8: Pour the base into a freezer-safe dish and freeze for an hour before whisking until smooth. Repeat this process 2-3 times, before stirring in the pecans and returning to the freezer.

*** The texture won't be exactly the same as when made with an ice cream maker, but it will still taste creamy and delicious ***

Apple Fritters – Paleo – Low Carb

Ingredients:

- ½ cup to 1 cup chopped apple
- ½ cup almond flour
- 2 tbsp. coconut flour
- 1 tbsp. white chia seeds
- ¼ cup coconut milk
- 3 tbsp. maple syrup
- 1 egg (cage free)
- ¾ tsp. ground cinnamon
- ¾ tsp. vanilla extract
- ½ tsp. baking soda
- 1 tsp. cream of tartar
- Pinch of sea salt
- 2 tbsp. coconut oil

Instructions:

Step 1: Preheat the oven to 350 degrees F.

Step 2: Dice the apple into small pieces and sauté over medium heat with a splash of coconut oil, ¼ teaspoon cinnamon, and ¼ teaspoon vanilla.

Step 3: Stir it frequently and cook until the apple is well cooked, for roughly 7 minutes. This will prevent uncooked spots around the apple pieces in the fritters.

Step 4: Mix all fritter ingredients together starting with almond flour and ending with a pinch of salt and then mix in the cooked apple pieces.

Step 5: Heat up a sauce pan over medium heat. Add in 2 tablespoons of coconut oil. When the oil is hot, spoon in a glob of dough to create a small chunky apple pancake. Try to keep the fritters on the smaller side so they are easy to manage and flip.

Step 6: Cook the fritters for about 1 to 2 minutes per side or until they are golden.

Step 7: The fritters will fall apart, but don't worry, just make them chunkier when cooking. After cooking each side for around 2 minutes, set each fritter on a baking sheet lined with parchment paper.

Step 8: After frying, bake the fritters for about 10 to 15 minutes at 350 degrees F.

*** While the fritters are baking prep the icing by following the recipe for the low carb icing ***

For the Low Carb Icing:

- ½ cup powdered erythritol
- 1 tbsp. coconut oil
- Splash of coconut milk
- ¼ tsp. vanilla powder
- Grind erythritol in a coffee grinder

Step 1: Mix powdered erythritol, goat milk butter, and vanilla powder in a bowl.

Step 2: Add a tiny splash of coconut milk at a time until you have the right consistency of icing.

Step 3: Drop chunks of icing over each fritter when they come out of the oven.

Cherry Paleo Milkshake

Ingredients:

For the Shake:

- 1 medium size banana
- ½ cup of pitted cherries
- Hint of vanilla extract
- 1 tbsp. chocolate chips (non-dairy)
- 1 cup dairy free milk

For the Whipped Topping:

- 2 tbsp. coconut cream

For the Magic Hardshell Chocolate Topping:

- 1 tsp. coconut oil
- 1 tsp. cocoa powder
- 1 tsp. honey

Instructions:

For the Shake:

Step 1: Place all ingredients in a magic bullet or blender and mix until smooth.

For the Whipped Topping:

Step 2: Place the coconut cream in a medium size bowl and whip with a hand mixer for 30 seconds to a minute, or until fluffy.

For the Magic Hardshell Chocolate:

Step 1: First, melt coconut oil, then add in cocoa powder and honey and mix until combined. The mixture should be drippy.

Step 2: When the mixture is poured on top of something cold, it will harden.

CONCLUSION:

I hope you have enjoyed reading this book and I hope that you will take the active steps to start your Paleo journey. There is nothing to be afraid of. The Paleo diet has many benefits for human health. These health benefits can take many forms, and a quick analysis of many Paleo diet discussions shows large groups of people who have had an improvement in their lives and health.

Start your Paleo diet today and start seeing a new and improved you.

Made in the USA
Monee, IL
10 April 2021

64783721R00114